Carcinogenesis Testing of Chemicals

Proceedings
CONFERENCE ON CARCINOGENESIS TESTING
IN THE DEVELOPMENT OF NEW DRUGS
May 23—25, 1973
Washington, D.C.

Editor

Leon Golberg, M.B., D.Phil., D.Sc.
President, Chemical Industry Institute of Toxicology
Research Triangle Park, North Carolina

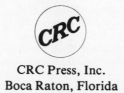

CRC Press, Inc.
Boca Raton, Florida

Library of Congress Cataloging in Publication Data

Conference on Carcinogenesis Testing in the Development
    of New Drugs, Washington, D.C., 1973.
    Carcinogenesis testing of chemicals.

    Includes bibliographies.
    1. Drugs — Testing — Congresses. 2. Chemicals —
Physiological effect — Congresses. 3. Carcinogenesis —
Congresses. I. Golberg, Leon, ed. II. Title.
[DNLM: 1. Carcinogens — Congresses. 2. Drug evalua-
tion — Congresses. 3. Drug screening — Congresses.
QZ202 C7472 1973]
RS189.C6122 1973   614.3'5   74-11693
ISBN 0-8493-5085-9

Direct all inquiries to CRC Press, 2000 N.W. 24th Street, Boca Raton, Florida, 33431.

© 1974 by CRC Press, Inc.
Second Printing, 1976
Third Printing, 1977
Fourth Printing, 1979
Fifth Printing, 1980

International Standard Book Number 0-8493-5085-9
Former International Standard Book Number 0-87819-058-9

Library of Congress Card Number 74-11693
Printed in the United States

PREFACE

Evaluation of drugs for carcinogenic potential is an essential aspect of drug development, yet difficult problems of science, ethics, and epidemiology surround this evaluation. Of particular interest is the question of the clinical relevance of carcinogenicity testing, and determinations in this area must rest upon a review of the present status of methodology as well as upon a determination of newer methods that may hold promise in carcinogenicity testing. The purpose of this Conference was to review both of these areas.

A number of individual papers were offered; however, the focus of the Conference was on the various discussion groups. Each of the latter prepared the summary reports that are included in this volume.

In 1915, Yamagiwa and Ichikawa demonstrated the carcinogenic property of coal tar by painting it repeatedly on the ears of rabbits. Their observations soon led to skin-painting tests for carcinogens in mice. From skin-painting it was a short step to the administration, by various routes, of compounds to common species of laboratory animals in life-span studies. This is essentially the current status of methodology; however, extensive application of these tests gradually led to the realization that, quite apart from the constituents of coal tar, a number of other chemical agents in common use were capable of inducing cancer in experimental animals. This led to the requirement that chemicals added to, and ingested in, food should be tested for carcinogenic potential by life-span studies in animals.

Even though the use of therapeutic agents, as compared with food additives, is more selective, better controlled, and — for the most part — more limited in duration, the need for carcinogenesis testing of drugs has become increasingly evident.

In 1966, the World Health Organization (WHO) set up a Scientific Group on Principles for Preclinical Testing of Drug Safety.[a] The report of this group contained some important generalizations, among which the following are instructive:

> "To be of maximum utility in allowing meaningful studies of drug safety to be performed, studies of drug metabolism must be carried out in man at an early stage of the drug's development . . . When all concerned are convinced that sufficient has been done to minimize the risk represented by a small number of controlled administrations to human beings, than absorption, metabolism and excretion of the drug should be studied in man, to a degree sufficient to permit a comprehensive study of toxicity in animals on a more rational basis. In particular, it should then be possible to choose species that resemble man in the way in which the drug is absorbed, distributed, metabolized, and excreted . . . The discussions have constantly stressed the need for an intelligent approach to the evaluation of the safety of a drug as a research problem in its own right, and this cannot be repeated too often. The application of all relevant new techniques to these problems must be actively encouraged even when their immediate usefulness cannot be seen clearly enough for them authoritatively to be recommended."

The report made reference to life-span toxicity studies, and on the subject of carcinogenicity it had this to say:

> "Assessment of a drug for carcinogenicity requires prolonged, detailed and exacting studies, the results of which are not always conclusive. Nevertheless, special attention should be given to carcinogenic assessment of compounds which are structurally related to known or suspected carcinogens and of drugs that affect mitosis or may be taken for a long time or are likely to be retained in the tissues."

Consideration of the question of carcinogenicity of drugs was taken further in 1968 by another WHO Scientific Group, which dealt specifically with Prinicples for the Testing and Evaluation of Drugs for Carcinogenicity. Certain parts of this report[b] are pertinent:

[a]*World Health Organization Technical Report*, No. 341, 1966.

[b]*World Health Organization Technical Report*, No. 426, 1969.

"Throughout this report, a distinction is drawn between testing a drug for carcinogenicity in animals and evaluating its carcinogenic hazard for man. Such evaluation may be based on the results of an experimental study in animals or on other information, such as the characteristics of the drug, the manner in which it is likely to be used, and epidemiological evidence. These considerations may indicate that the experimental studies in animals are unnecessary for a given drug . . . The possibility of carcinogenic hazard, and therefore the need for assessment in this respect, exist in relation to all drugs. Confident prediction of the carcinogenicity or noncarcinogenicity of a given drug is not possible on the basis of its chemical structure or biological activity, although such properties may indicate that high priority should be given to the testing of a given product."

The report then went on to set priorities for testing for carcinogenic potential, which may be summarized as follows:

1. Drugs to be tested before they are given to man.
   a. Drugs chemically related to known carcinogens.
   b. Drugs with certain specific biological effects (for instance, damage to rapidly growing tissues or effects on mitosis).
2. Drugs to be tested during clinical trial (e.g., those likely to be administered for prolonged periods or to newborn babies and pregnant or lactating women).
3. Drugs to be tested after the decision to release for marketing.
4. Drugs on the market that should be tested.

As more and more of the existing drugs came to be tested for their capacity to induce tumors in experimental animals, some very important and valuable therapeutic agents were indeed found to possess this capacity. Even though in most instances there was no indication of corresponding effects in man, it became clear that fresh consideration should be given to the timing of tests for carcinogenicity with respect to new medicines. Ideally, such tests should be completed before any human exposure to the compound takes place. In practice, however, until there is some idea of human absorption, metabolism, and disposition of a drug, it is difficult, if not impossible, to determine the relevance to man of carcinogenicity studies in particular species of animals. Even more importantly, it may be said in general that, at that early stage, no decision can be reached concerning the relative merits or even usefulness of any one of a series of likely candidate compounds.

Given this situation, therefore, two separate and distinct needs exist:

1. Short-term tests that may be used as reliable indicators of lack of carcinogenic potential. Such tests may thus be applied before Phase I studies are undertaken in man.

2. Improvements in the existing procedures for life-span tests of carcinogenicity. This need has been discussed on many occasions in recent years, notably by the Panel on Carcinogenesis of the Food and Drug Administration's Advisory Committee on Protocols for Safety Evaluation. This Panel served under the chairmanship of Dr. Philip Shubik, and its report was published in *Toxicology and Applied Pharmacology*, 20, 419, 1971.

The present Conference was organized for the purpose of approaching these issues.* Four topics were considered:

1. The present state-of-the-art in carcinogenesis testing, using currently accepted procedures to identify potential carcinogens.

2. Tests already proposed for identification of potential carcinogens, or tests that could be developed for this purpose on the basis of existing knowledge.

*The Committee responsible for the organization of the Conference included Dr. Daniel L. Azarnoff, Dr. Bernard B. Brodie, Dr. William D'Aguanno, Dr. James R. Gillette, Dr. Leon Golberg (Chairman), Dr. Arthur P. Grollman, and Dr. Harold M. Perk. Dr. Joseph A. DiPaolo and Dr. Umberto Saffiotti were consultants to the Committee. The Editor's sincere thanks are due to the members and consultants for their sterling efforts.

3. Monitoring of patients who were exposed to drugs that are later found to produce tumors in experimental animals.

4. Ethical considerations that are involved at present in human exposure to new drugs.

As plans for the Conference developed, attention was confined to the first two of these topics, emphasizing the need to take stock of present thinking on procedures for life-span studies and on possible new approaches to carcinogenesis testing.

In developing plans for the present Conference, the Ad Hoc Subcommittee confined its attention to the first two of these questions, emphasizing the need to take stock of present thinking on procedures for life-span studies and on possible new approaches to carcinogenesis testing.

There is some hesitation to apply the newer procedures. Feelings about the newer tests may be summed up in Sir Winston Churchill's comment on a member of the House of Commons named Bossom: "He's neither the one thing nor the other." Applying the new procedures is neither research nor formal testing, and some ground rules are needed if the resources and expertise of the pharmaceutical industry are to be brought to bear on the exploration of the new techniques.

The Conference had a somewhat unusual structure. Fifteen discussion groups were set up in advance, each under its own leader, and these met for an entire day on May 23, 1973, to prepare reports and recommendations in specific areas falling within the two main lines of inquiry. On May 24 and 25, the respective leaders of the discussion groups presented their reports to the plenary session, the subject matter having been organized in such fashion that currently accepted procedures were discussed on May 24 and newer approaches on May 25. This volume incorporates the majority of the reports of the discussion groups.

In a number of instances, working papers had been prepared and circulated to the members of the respective discussion groups, so that the salient, and possibly contentious, issues could be clarified in advance of the Conference. This arrangement enjoyed considerable success and acceptance among the discussion groups. The 15 groups, together with others attending the Conference, engaged in keen and productive analysis of the problems in the areas with which they were concerned. The reports of the discussion groups are valuable distillates of the current state-of-the-art in their respective fields.

Two of the reports of the discussion groups require special comment. The report on Inception and Duration of Tests (Discussion Group No. 4) recommends that life-span studies be carried on for 24 months in the case of mice and 30 months in the case of rats. It recommends further that: "no test be accepted as negative unless a statistically significant proportion of the test animals survive" for these periods. In practice, most laboratories — commercial, industrial, or academic — would find it virtually impossible to achieve such longevity in a sufficient proportion of treated, or even of control, animals. Hence, it is suggested by the Conference Chairman, Dr. Leon Golberg, that the duration of studies required for regulatory purposes — 18 months for mice and 24 months for rats — remain an attainable and adequate standard.

The use of positive controls in carcinogenicity studies also requires comment. Two sections in this volume are devoted to this controversial question. The second of these, entitled "Positive Controls in Environmental Respiratory Carcinogenesis" and authored by D. Hoffmann and E. L. Wynder, was not presented at the Conference, but it is included here in order to illustrate the value of positive controls in bioassays for carcinogens. It should be stressed, however, that the subject of the Conference was the testing of *drugs*, and in the case of drugs the question to which a clear and unequivocal answer is needed is altogether different from the problem of tobacco carcinogenesis — the problem with which Drs. Hoffman and Wynder are largely concerned. Drs. J. H. and E. K. Weisburger have provided a report on positive control carcinogens in standardized in vivo and in vitro carcinogen bioassay procedures that makes a case for the use of positive controls, but the report concludes that "specifically in relation to the bioassay of drugs, omission of a contemporary positive control series may be permissible." A substantial proportion of those engaged in safety-testing of drugs would agree, in Dr. Golberg's view, that the use of positive controls should remain optional.

The first paper of the Conference, "Design of Experiments to Detect Carcinogenic Effects of Drugs," was presented by Dr. Harold M. Peck. His paper originated from a working paper prepared as a guide in the discussions that ultimately led to the decision to organize the present Conference. Thus, the contents differ in format from that usually expected in a review paper or in a presentation involving a detailed discussion of methodology. The paper is, rather, an attempt to coordinate the experimental procedures used by oncologists and toxicologists, recognizing the different specific needs of each group while also recognizing that the ultimate goal of both groups is the demonstration of carcinogenicity or non-carcinogenicity of a chemical agent.

ACKNOWLEDGMENT

The Conference was supported by the Food and Drug Administration under Contract No. FDA 70-22, Task Order 18, by the National Cancer Institute under Contract No. PH43-64-44, Task Order 69, by the National Institute of General Medical Sciences under Contract No. PH43-NIGMS-64-44, Task Order 5, and by a Grant from the Pharmaceutical Manufacturers Association Foundation, Inc.

THE EDITOR

Leon Golberg was born in Cyprus and attended the University of the Witwatersrand, Johannesburg, where he majored in Mathematics and Chemistry. He was awarded the William Cullen Medal (for the best graduate in Science) and obtained First Class Honours in Organic Chemistry. Proceeding to a Master's degree in Physical Chemistry, he was awarded an Overseas Fellowship that enabled him to work under Sir Robert Robinson at Oxford. There he participated in the synthetic effort that culminated in the discovery of stilbestrol and related estrogens. After completing his D.Phil., he was awarded the Cornwall and York Prize by the Vice-Chancellors' Committee of the South African Universities and a Fellowship by the Medical Research Council of Great Britain.

Shortly after his return to the Chemistry Department at the University of the Witwatersrand, the outbreak of World War II caused Dr. Golberg to undertake defense-related biochemical research at the South African Institute for Medical Research, where he remained until 1946. His biochemical investigations culminated in the award of the D.Sc. degree by the University of the Witwatersrand.

Returning to England, Dr. Golberg embarked on preclinical studies in Cambridge, where he was elected Senior Scholar of Emmanuel College and was awarded the Colin Mackenzie, Albert Hopkinson, and Emmanuel College prizes. Clinical experience was gained at University College Hospital Medical School and at Addenbrook's Hospital, Cambridge. Appointed Senior Lecturer in Chemical Pathology in the Department of Pathology at the University of Manchester, Dr. Golberg carried out research on artherosclerosis and on inborn errors of metabolism, notably galactosemia. In 1955 he joined Benger Laboratories Ltd. (now Fisons Pharmaceuticals Ltd.) as Medical Research Director and engaged in investigations of iron metabolism, the biochemical and pathological consequences of iron overloading, and subcutaneous sarcoma produced in rodents by iron dextran. When the British Industrial Biological Research Association (BIBRA) was formed in 1961, Dr. Golberg was appointed Director. He started *BIBRA Bulletin*, and founded and edited *Food and Cosmetics Toxicology*. After six years of research on food-additive toxicology, subcutaneous carcinogenesis and the biochemical aspects of liver enlargement, Dr. Golberg was invited by the Royal College of Physicians of London to deliver the Milroy Lectures. He was also a Founder Fellow of the Royal College of Pathologists. In 1967 he accepted an invitation to become Scientific Director and Research Professor of Pathology at the Institute of Experimental Pathology and Toxicology, Albany Medical College, in Albany, N.Y.

In America, Dr. Golberg has been active in research as well as in training in Toxicology. He has continued to serve as Consultant to the World Health Organization, and has served the Food and Drug Administration, the National Institutes of Health, and the National Academy of Sciences in various capacities. In 1969 he was Chairman of the Subcommittee on Effects of Pesticides on Man of the Secretary's (of HEW) Commission on Pesticides and Their Relationship to Environmental Health.

Dr. Golberg is a member of the Scientific Advisory Board of the National Center for Toxicological Research and of the Hazardous Materials Advisory Committee of the Environmental Protection Agency. Amoung other editorial activities, he is Editor of *CRC Critical Reviews in Toxicology* and of the Uniscience Series of Monographs in Toxicology.

Dr. Golberg has been president of the Chemical Industry Institute of Toxicology at Research Triangle Park, North Carolina, since Febuary, 1976.

CONTRIBUTORS

Robert K. Bickerton, Ph.D.
Department of Pharmacology
Norwich Pharmacal Company
Norwich, New York

David B. Clayson, Ph.D.
School of Medicine
University of Leeds
Leeds, Yorkshire, England

William D'Aguanno, Ph.D.
Division of Neuropharmacology
Bureau of Drugs
Food and Drug Administration
Rockville, Maryland

Frederick J. deSerres, Ph.D.
Biology Division
Oak Ridge National Laboratory
Oak Ridge Tennessee

Joseph A. DiPaolo, Ph.D.
Cytogenetics and Cytology Section
National Cancer Institute
National Institutes of Health
Bethesda, Maryland

Joseph F. Fraumeni, Jr., M.D.
Epidemiology Branch
National Cancer Institute
National Institutes of Health
Bethesda, Maryland

Aaron E. Freeman, Ph.D.
Microbial Associates, Inc.
Bethesda, Maryland

Leo Friedman, Ph.D. (deceased)
Division of Toxicology
Bureau of Foods
Food and Drug Administration
Rockville, Maryland

Leon Golberg, M.B., D.Phil., D.Sc., F.R.C. Path.
President
Chemical Industry Institute of Toxicology
Research Triangle Park, North Carolina

Dietrich Hoffmann, Ph.D.
Naylor Dana Institute for Disease Prevention
American Health Foundation
New York, New York

Daniel Nebert, M.D.
Developmental Pharmacology
National Institute of Child Health and Human
  Development
National Institutes of Health
Bethesda, Maryland

Paul M. Newberne, Ph.D.
Department of Nutrition and Food Science
Massachusetts Institute of Technology
Cambridge, Massachusetts

Harold M. Peck, M.D.
Department of Safety Assessment
Merck Institute for Therapeutic Research
Merck, Sharpe & Dohme Research Laboratories
West Point, Pennsylvania

Henry C. Pitot, M.D., Ph.D.
McArdle Laboratory
School of Medicine
University of Wisconsin
Madison, Wisconsin

David P. Rall, M.D., Ph.D.
National Institute of Environmental Health
  Sciences
Research Triangle Park, North Carolina

Melvin D. Reuber, M.D.
Department of Pathology
School of Medicine
University of Maryland
Baltimore, Maryland

D. S. R. Sarma, Ph.D.
Fels Research Institute
Temple University
Philadelphia, Pennsylvania

Michal B. Shimkin, M.D.
Department of Community Medicine
School of Medicine
University of California at San Diego
La Jolla, California

Philippe Shubik, M.D., Ph.D.
Eppley Institute for Research in Cancer
University of Nebraska
Omaha, Nebraska

L. Tomatis, M.D.
World Health Organization
Lyon, France

Bernard Weinstein, M.D.
Institute of Cancer Research
Columbia University
New York, New York

John H. Weisburger, Ph.D.
Vice President for Research
American Health Foundation
New York, New York

Ernest L. Wynder, M.D.
President and Medical Director
American Health Foundation
New York, New York

ROSTER OF MEMBERS OF
DISCUSSION GROUPS

DISCUSSION GROUP NO. 1
Species and Strain Selection
Leader:
Dr. Michal B. Shimkin
Members:
Dr. Thomas Cameron
  Program Data Analysis Unit
  National Institutes of Health
  Bethesda, Maryland
Dr. Norbert Page
  Head, Program Data and Analysis Unit
  National Institutes of Health
  Bethesda, Maryland
Dr. J. D. Prejean
  Head, Chemical Carcinogenesis Section
  Southern Research Institute
  Birmingham, Alabama
Dr. Gary D. Stoner
  Assistant Research Scientist
  University of California School of Medicine
  La Jolla, California
Dr. D. Jane Taylor
  Head, Experimental Biology Project Section
  Breast Cancer Program
  National Institutes of Health
  Bethesda, Maryland

DISCUSSION GROUP NO. 2
Diets
Leader:
Dr. Paul M. Newberne
Members:
Dr. John G. Bieri
  Chief, Nutrition and Biochemistry Section
  National Institute of Arthritis, Metabolism, and
    Digestive Diseases
  National Institutes of Health
  Bethesda, Maryland
Dr. Colin Campbell
  Department of Biochemistry and Nutrition
  Virginia Polytechnic Institute and State University
  Blacksburg, Virginia
Dr. Lionel Poirier
  National Cancer Institute
  National Institutes of Health
  Bethesda, Maryland
Dr. Adrianne E. Rogers
  Senior Research Scientist
  Massachusetts Institute of Technology
  Cambridge, Massachusetts
Dr. Maurice Shils
  Attending Physician
  Memorial Hospital
  New York, New York

Dr. Lee Wattenberg
  Professor of Pathology
  University of Minnesota Medical School
  Minneapolis, Minnesota

DISCUSSION GROUP NO. 3
Dose Selection and Administration
Leader:
Dr. Leo Friedman
Members:
Dr. Bert J. Bos
  Medical Director
  Woodard Research Corp.
  Herndon, Virginia
Dr. James M. Price
  Vice President, Abbott Laboratories
  Corporation Research and Experimental Therapy
  North Chicago, Illinois
Dr. Gerald N. Wogan
  Professor of Toxicology
  Massachusetts Institute of Technology
  Cambridge, Massachusetts

DISCUSSION GROUP NO. 4
Inception and Duration of Tests
Leader:
Dr. L. Tomatis
Members:
Dr. R. Montesano
  Unit of Chemical Carcinogenesis
  IARC World Health Organization
  Lyon, France
Dr. Jerry Rice
  Experimental Pathology Branch
  National Cancer Institute
  National Institutes of Health
  Bethesda, Maryland
Dr. Stan Vesselinovitch
  Radiology
  University of Chicago
  Chicago, Illinois

DISCUSSION GROUP NO. 5
Inclusion of Positive Control Compounds
Leader:
Dr. John H. Weisburger
Members:
Dr. Dietrich Hoffmann
  Naylor Dana Institute for Disease Prevention
    of the American Health Foundation
  New York, New York

Dr. James M. Price
  Vice President, Abbott Laboratories
  Corporation Research and Experimental Therapy
  North Chicago, Illinois
Participants:
Dr. Saul Bader,
  Pharmacologist
  Division of Oncology
  Food and Drug Administration
  Rockville, Maryland
Dr. David Clayson
  Professor of Pathology (Visiting)
  University of Nebraska
  Omaha, Nebraska

Dr. J. M. Davitt
  Pharmacologist
  Bureau of Drugs
  Food and Drug Administration
  Rockville, Maryland
Dr. R. M. Diener
  Director, Toxicology and Pathology
  Ciba-Geigy Corporation
  Summit, New Jersey
Dr. Ruth Kirschstein
  Deputy Assistant Commissioner for Science
  Food and Drug Administration
  Rockville, Maryland
Dr. Harold M. Peck
  Director, Department of Safety Assessment
  Merck, Sharpe & Dohme
  West Point, Pennsylvania
Dr. John J. Pollock
  Director, Animal Health Division
  Ayerst Research Laboratories
  Chazy, New York
Dr. Robert McConnell
  Director, Department of Pathology-Toxicology
  G. D. Searle & Co.
  Chicago, Illinois
Dr. Edward Schwartz
  Director, Department of Toxicology
  Warner-Lambert Research Institute
  Morris Plains, New Jersey
Dr. Robert Zwicky
  Associate Director, Department of Safety
    Assessment
  Merck, Sharpe & Dohme
  West Point, Pennsylvania

DISUCSSION GROUP NO. 7
Spontaneous Tumors and Related Pathologic
  Changes
Leader:
Dr. R. K. Bickerton

Members:
Dr. Raymond B. Baggs
  New England Regional Primate Research Center
  Harvard Medical School
  Southboro, Massachusetts
Dr. Thelma Dunn
  National Cancer Institute
  National Institutes of Health
  Bethesda, Maryland
Dr. Margaret K. Deringer
  National Cancer Institute
  National Institutes of Health
  Bethesda, Maryland
Dr. Katherine Snell
  National Cancer Institute
  National Institutes of Health
  Bethesda, Maryland
Dr. Harold L. Stewart
  National Cancer Institute
  National Institutes of Health
  Bethesda, Maryland
Dr. Richard L. Swarm
  Experimental Pathology and Toxicology
  Hoffman-La Roche
  Nutley, New Jersey
Dr. Samuel W. Thompson
  Pathology Department
  CIBA Pharmaceutical Company
  Summit, New Jersey

DISCUSSION GROUP NO. 8
Criteria for Tumor Diagnosis and Classification of
  Malignancy
Leader:
Dr. Melvin D. Reuber
Members:
Dr. Borge Ulland
  Frederick Cancer Research Center
  Frederick, Maryland
Dr. Jerry Ward
  National Cancer Institute
  National Institutes of Health
  Bethesda, Maryland

DISCUSSION GROUP NO. 10
Metabolic Activation as Factor in Carcinogenic
  Response
Leader:
Dr. Daniel Nebert
Members:
Dr. Bruce N. Ames
  Professor of Biochemistry
  University of California
  Berkeley, California

Dr. Donald M. Jerina
  National Institute of Arthritis, Metabolism,
    and Digestive Diseases
  National Institutes of Health
  Bethesda, Maryland
Dr. K. Lemone
  Director of the Laboratory of Molecular
    Biology
  University of Alabama Medical Center
  Birmingham, Alabama
Dr. Snorri Thorgeirsson
  National Heart and Lung Institute
  National Institutes of Health
  Bethesda, Maryland
Dr. Irene Y. Wang
  Cancer Research Institute
  University of California
  San Francisco, California

DISCUSSION GROUP NO. 11
Chemical Interaction Measurements
Leader:
Dr. D. S. R. Sarma
Members:
Dr. Earl Bayliss
  Sloane Kettering Institute
  New York, New York
Dr. Jay I. Goodman
  Department of Pharmacology
  Michigan State University
  East Lansing, Michigan
Dr. H. F. Stich
  Professor of Genetics
  Cancer Research Center
  University of British Columbia
  Vancouver, B.C., Canada

DISCUSSION GROUP NO. 12
Mutagenesis Assessment
Leader:
Dr. Frederick J. deSerres
Members:
Dr. Ernest Chu
  Department of Human Genetics
  University of Michigan Medical School
  Ann Arbor, Michigan
Dr. Frank H. Mukai
  Department of Environmental Medicine
  New York University Medical Center
  New York, New York
Dr. Lionel Poirier
  National Cancer Institute
  National Institutes of Health
  Bethesda, Maryland

Dr. Hans W. Ruelies
  Manager, Metabolism Chemistry Section
  Wayeth Laboratories
  Philadelphia, Pennsylvania

DISCUSSION GROUP NO. 13
Tissue Culture Technics
Leader:
Dr. Bernard Weinstein
Members:
Dr. Charles Evans
  National Cancer Institute
  National Institutes of Health
  Bethesda, Maryland
Dr. Charles Heidelberger
  McArdle Laboratory
  University of Wisconsin
  Madison, Wisconsin
Dr. Andrew Sivak
  Department of Environmental Medicine
  New York University Medical School
  New York, New York
Dr. Michael Sporn
  National Cancer Institute
  National Institutes of Health
  Bethesda, Maryland

DISCUSSION GROUP NO. 14
Criteria of Neoplastic Transformation
Leader:
Dr. Henry C. Pitot
Members:
Dr. Peter Nowell
  Department of Pathology
  University of Pennsylvania School of Medicine
  Philadelphia, Pennsylvania
Dr. G. Barry Pierce
  Department of Pathology
  University of Colorado Medical Center
  Denver, Colorado
Dr. Richmond Prehn
  Institute for Cancer Research
  Philadelphia, Pennsylvania

DISCUSSION GROUP NO. 15
Problems of Development of Systems with
  Materials of Human Origin
Leader:
Dr. Aaron Freeman
Members:
Dr. T. Timothy Crocker
  University of California College of Medicine
  Irvine, California

Dr. Leila Diamond
  Wistar Institute
  Philadelphia, Pennsylvania
Dr. Leonard Hayflick
  Stanford University School of Medicine
  Stanford, California
Dr. Howard Igel
  Children's Hospital
  Akron, Ohio

Dr. Richard Kouri
  Microbiological Associates, Inc.
  Bethesda, Maryland
Dr. Bernard Lane
  State University of New York
  Stoneybrook, New York
Dr. Paul Price
  Microbiological Associates, Inc.
  Bethesda, Maryland

TABLE OF CONTENTS

Section 1
Design of Experiments to Detect Carcinogenic Effect of Drugs 1
Harold M. Peck

Section 2
Species and Strain Selection. Report of Discussion Group No. 1 15
Michael B. Shimkin

Section 3
Diets. Report of Discussion Group No. 2 17
Paul M. Newberne

Section 4
Dose Selection and Administration. Report of Discussion Group No. 3 21
Leo Friedman

Section 5
Inception and Duration of Tests. Report of Discussion Group No. 4 23
L. Tomatis

Section 6
Inclusion of Positive Control Compounds. Report of Discussion Group No. 5 29
John H. Weisburger

Section 7
Positive Controls in Environmental Respiratory Carcinogens 35
Dietrich Hoffmann and Ernest L. Wynder

Section 8
Interpretation of Test Results in Terms of Carcinogenic Potential to the Test Animal: The Regulatory Point
of View 41
William D'Aguanno

Section 9
Interpretation of Test Results in Terms of Significance to Man 45
Philippe Shubik

Section 10
Carcinogenic Effects of Drugs in Man 51
Joseph F. Fraumeni, Jr.

Section 11
Spontaneous Tumors and Related Pathologic Changes. Report of Discussion Group No. 7 . . . , . . 55
R. K. Bickerton

Section 12
Criteria for Tumor Diagnosis and Classification of Malignancy. Report of Discussion Group No. 8 . . 71
Melvin Reuber

Section 13
Metabolic Activation as a Factor in Carcinogenic Response. Report of Discussion Group No. 10 . . . 75
Daniel Nebert

Section 14
Historical Evolution of Short-Term Tests for Carcinogenicity 79
David B. Clayson

Section 15
Short-Term Tests for Carcinogenesis: Tests Involving Induction of Neoplasia 91
J. A. DiPaolo

Section 16
Chemical Interaction Measurements. Report of Discussion Group No. 11 95
D. S. R. Sarma

Section 17
Mutagenesis Assessment. Report of Discussion Group No. 12 101
Frederick J. de Serres

Section 18
Tissue Culture Techniques. Report of Discussion Group No. 13 109
Bernard Weinstein

Section 19
Criteria of Neoplastic Transformation. Report of Discussion Group No. 14 113
Henry C. Pitot

Section 20
Problems of Development of Systems with Materials of Human Origin. Report of Discussion Group No. 15 115
Aaron Freeman

Section 21
Summary and Concluding Remarks 119
David P. Rall

Section 22
Recommendations of the Conference as Stated by the Conference Chairman 123
Leon Golberg

Index 125

SECTION 1
DESIGN OF EXPERIMENTS TO DETECT CARCINOGENIC EFFECTS OF DRUGS

Harold M. Peck

Experiments to detect the potential carcinogenic effects of drugs can be considered to be modifications of the chronic toxicology studies commonly done in many laboratories. In essence, the procedure is to treat animals with the drug for the "life span" of the animal to determine if there are differences in the time of appearance and in the number and types of tumors between treated animals and controls. The rat and the mouse are usually used in carcinogenic studies, since they are known to be sensitive to many of the known carcinogenic agents, have a relatively short life span, and are commonly used in the laboratory for pharmacology and toxicology studies. Nonrodents, such as the dog and monkey, are seldom used because of their long life span[8,32,34] and the impracticality of using the large numbers desirable for statistical purposes.

Because the life-span studies require a large expenditure of time, space and manpower, a number of investigators have been searching for short-term carcinogenic tests that would provide rapid and reliable detection of the carcinogenic potential of chemicals and drugs. These methods include exposure of the fetus *in utero,* treating newborn animals, implanting treated embryonic tissue into a host of the same species,[23,24] tissue and organ culture techniques, microbiological techniques, and others.[4,32] It has been suggested that chemicals giving positive results in teratogenic and mutagenic tests will also be carcinogenic. Unfortunately, a positive correlation is not obtained with sufficient consistency to permit acceptance of these techniques for determining carcinogenic potential. Much more research using such experimental procedures, including agreement with the results of life-span studies in animals and with agents known to be carcinogenic for man, is required before these techniques can be substituted for the life-span studies. Since the short-term tests are not yet acceptable as a substitute, it is appropriate to examine the experimental procedure available to the toxicologist — the life-span experiments in rodents. This procedure has been used for many years to detect potential carcinogenic properties of those chemicals to be used in foods that are under no suspicion, or only vague suspicion, of carcinogenic potential.

The following discussion will be concerned with the suggested procedures for study of such chemicals. An excellent discussion of carcinogenic studies presented by Weisburger and Weisburger in *Methods in Cancer Research*[32] is recommended for study.

Very briefly, the experimental design for carcinogenic testing in the life-span study is as follows:

Each treated group and control group of animals should consist of enough males and females of the desired species and strain to provide an adequate number of survivors at the termination of the experiment to permit pathologic and statistical evaluations (Table 1). Two or three dose levels of the chemical are used, the highest being that which can be tolerated without toxicity. The low dose level is usually selected to be some multiple of the exposure level for man. The animals are weighed periodically and observed frequently for tumor development (Table 2). The route of administration is usually the same as that to be used in man. Animals dying or killed during the study are examined at autopsy to determine the cause of death and presence of tumors, and histopathologic studies are done as indicated. At termination all animals are examined grossly and a selected number of high-dose and control animals are examined microscopically; target organs from all animals are also examined microscopically. Each of these points will be discussed in more detail.

SELECTION OF TEST ANIMALS

The strains of rats and mice to be used in carcinogenic studies of drugs may be the same strains used in the pharmacology and toxicology evaluation of drugs. This is useful because the activity of the drug in those strains is known and the selection of appropriate dose levels can be made without additional studies. The rats and mice most commonly used in the toxicology

TABLE 1

Outline of Experiment for Carcinogenic Testing in the Rodent

	Number of animals in each dose group			
	Control	Low	Middle	High
Male	25 to 50	25 to 50	25 to 50	25 to 50
Female	25 to 50	25 to 50	25 to 50	25 to 50
Total	200 to 400 (preferred)			
Proposed duration	Rats – 24 months Mice – 18 months			

TABLE 2

Outline of Experiment for Carcinogenic Testing in the Rodent

Food consumption (if drug given in diet)	Weekly for 12 weeks Monthly for duration
Body weight	Weekly for 12 weeks Monthly for duration
Observations	At least weekly, especially for tumor development; hematology if leukemia suspected
Gross pathology	All deaths and sacrifices
Histopathology	Partial or complete or all deaths (if post-mortem changes not too advanced), and sacrifices prior to termination Complete on control and high dose at termination Target organs – all animals Tissues with gross lesions of uncertain character

experiments are outbred (random-bred) strains and in many cases have been shown to be sensitive to carcinogenic agents. Each laboratory would have, and is continually collecting, historical and concurrent background data of spontaneous-tumor incidence from control animals used in toxicology and carcinogenic studies. Both historical and concurrent control data should be used for evaluating tumor incidence in treated animals.

The question of the strain of animal to be used needs to be finally resolved. The trend appears to be toward acceptance of the outbred strains.[8,33] These strains may have a variable, moderately high incidence of specific types of tumors and in addition usually have a low incidence of other types of tumors. Inbred strains may have a

constant and relatively high incidence of a specific tumor, i.e., lung, liver or mammary, and a low incidence of other types of tumors.

If a chemical is known to induce the type of tumor found in high incidence in an inbred strain of rodent, the oncologist has used that inbred strain to study structurally similar compounds and the mechanism of carcinogenicity.[34] This would appear to be a logical procedure. If a new drug has a structure similar to that of a known carcinogen, an appropriate inbred strain might be used, although the toxicologist knows that predicting toxicity on the basis of structure is not always reliable. However, if the structure of a drug is not similar to that of a known carcinogen, there is no way of knowing which, if any, tumor that drug might induce, and therefore it would be impossible to select an appropriate inbred strain of mouse or rat from the many strains available. It has been stated that "The ideal strain would be one with no incidence of spontaneous tumors and a high general susceptibility to carcinogenic agents."[34]

NUMBER OF ANIMALS

The number of animals suggested for use in carcinogenic studies is 25 to 50 males and 25 to 50 females in the control group and in each drug-treated group. The larger number is more appropriate, since so many deaths may occur during the experiment, due to infections, spontaneous-tumor development and other causes, that meaningful statistical analysis at the termination of the experiment may be difficult. Proper random distribution of animals in cages, and possibly littermate distribution by sex across all groups, has been suggested as a means of decreasing the group variations of death and spontaneous-tumor development due to environmental and genetic factors. If the number of deaths is great enough, it may be desirable to terminate the study early, so that valid pathologic and statistical evaluations may be made. However, animal husbandry has improved so much that the problem of deaths due to spontaneous infections is not as great as it has been in the past.

Because of the variation in incidence of spontaneous tumors, the statisticians would prefer that the number of control animals be increased. Some laboratories are partially satisfying the desire for a larger number of control animals by using two control groups, each equal in number to one treated group. This is useful because the tumor incidence between the control groups can be compared, each control group can be compared with each treated group, or the control groups can be combined for comparison with the treated groups.

Some statisticians would like to have larger numbers of animals used in each group; groups of thousands have been mentioned. The value of using such large numbers of animals must be weighed against the overall cost and manpower requirements and the statistical benefit. There is some question whether increasing the number of animals from 100 to 500 per group would be of proportionate value in predicting risk; although there may be a statistical difference, biologically the difference may not be important (Tables 3A and 3B).

DOSAGE LEVELS

Two or three dosage levels are used in the carcinogenic studies. The highest dose may be the largest amount tolerated without observable toxic effects, including depressed growth rate or decreased food intake, as determined in toxicity studies of 3 to 12 months' duration. The WHO Scientific Group on Carcinogenesis, however, suggested that the highest dose should be within the toxic range if it is compatible with prolonged survival of most of the animals.[35] The lowest dosage level for drugs should be near the therapeutic dose for man. If a third dose level is used, it is selected to be about midway between the high and the low dosage levels.

TABLE 3A

Smallest Statistically Significant Percentage of Animals with Tumors on a Drug Dose (P_D) Compared to Animals with Varying Percentages of Tumors on Control (P_C). Based on Fisher's Exact Test at $P \leqslant 0.05$ (One-sided)

% with tumors on controls (P_C)	Number of animals on		% with tumors on drug dose (P_D)
	Controls	Drug dose	
0	50	50	10
	100	50	6
	500	50	4
10	50	50	26
	100	50	22
	500	50	20
20	50	50	38
	100	50	34
	500	50	32
30	50	50	50
	100	50	46
	500	50	44
40	50	50	60
	100	50	56
	500	50	54
50	50	50	70
	100	50	66
	500	50	64

Courtesy J. L. Ciminera.

Smallest Statistically Significant Percentage of Animals with Tumors on a Drug Dose (P_D) Compared to Animals with Varying Percentages of Tumors on Control (P_C). Based on Fisher's Exact Test at $P \leqslant 0.05$ (Two-sided)

% with tumors on controls (P_C)	Number of animals on		% with tumors on drug dose (P_D)
	Controls	Drug dose	
0	50	50	12
	100	100	6
	500	500	4
10	50	50	28
	100	100	21
	500	500	15
20	50	50	40
	100	100	34
	500	500	26
30	50	50	52
	100	100	45
	500	500	37
40	50	50	62
	100	100	55
	500	500	47
50	50	50	72
	100	100	65
	500	500	57

Courtesy J. L. Ciminera.

The therapeutic dose for man cannot always be used as a basis for animal studies. Occasionally a drug is more toxic for animals than for man. In contrast, occasionally a drug can be tolerated by animals at levels many times the pharmacologically active dose for man. The selection of dose levels for each drug must be based upon the known biological activity of that agent and the probable human exposure.

DOSE–RESPONSE

If a dose–response curve is to be obtained, the doses should be sufficiently spread so that an adequate dose-related response can be obtained. Since the validity of a dose–response curve with extrapolation to a "no effect" carcinogenic level is not generally accepted,[15,16,18] it is questionable whether more than two dose levels are necessary. However, a good dose–response curve using three dose levels might permit a better evaluation of potential risk if the drug is sufficiently valuable for use in spite of demonstration of carcinogenicity for animals.[4] The interpretation of a dose–response curve and the possibility of a "no effect" carcinogenic level need to be explored to determine if they are meaningful.[31] The refusal to accept a "no effect" level seems to be based upon the lack of ability to prove the absence of such an effect statistically and upon the proposition that alteration of one cell by one molecule is all that is needed to produce cancer.

ROUTE OF ADMINISTRATION

The route of administration in carcinogenic studies, as in toxicology studies, should be the same as the exposure route for man.[4] It has been suggested that parenteral as well as oral routes be used. However, it seems illogical to use the parenteral route in animals when the human exposure is oral, since the metabolism of a drug given parenterally may be different than when given by the oral route.[31]

Injecting a drug into the subcutaneous tissue of rats and mice is not a good procedure, because the physical and chemical characteristics of the material being injected may cause sufficient appropriate irritation to produce local subcutaneous tumors.[13,14,25] The rodents are particularly susceptible to materials injected in this manner, and certainly local tumors due to local irritant effects bear no relevancy to oral administration, although the induction of tumors in other sites might be meaningful.

If drugs are to be used parenterally in man (intravenous, subcutaneous, etc.), these routes should also be used in animals. It is difficult, if not impossible, to administer the drug daily to rats and mice for months by these routes, particularly if the drug has even minimal irritancy. The possibility of weekly or even less frequent injections, or treatment for a few weeks followed by observation for a total of 18 months in mice and 24 months in rats might be considered. If the metabolism of the drug by the parenteral routes is the same as by oral administration, the latter route might be substituted for the carcinogenic studies.

DURATION

The duration of carcinogenic studies may be established as 18 months for mice and 24 months for rats. This is a more logical designation of the duration than the term "life span," which could be taken to mean the average life span of the rodent or survival to death of each animal.

The duration should be flexible enough to permit early termination in the event of excessively reduced numbers of survivors, provided that the greater part of the proposed duration of the experiment has been completed. It is more important to have a shortened study with an adequate number of surviving animals to permit good statistical and pathologic evaluations than to have too few animals for these purposes. If an agent is a potent, or moderately potent, carcinogen, this may be determined prior to the proposed termination of the carcinogenic study, and the carcinogenic potential may be found in the course of the toxicology studies.[5] Several reports of toxicologic and carcinogenic studies reveal that carcinogenic effects in animals were detected when the agent was given for 12 months or less.[1,3,11, 20-22,26,29,32]

If a drug is to be given for a short period of time, such as three months to man, a period of three months' administration to animals and the observation of the animals for the remainder of the experimental period should be adequate. On the other hand, long-term continuous administration should reveal any carcinogenic potential earlier than by using the short administration period followed by a long period of observation, because the time of onset of tumor induction is apparently proportional to the duration of exposure and the total dose over that period of time.

PATHOLOGY

The procedure suggested for pathology studies of animals used in carcinogenic studies is similar to those used for toxicology studies and was discussed in the report of the WHO Scientific Group on Carcinogenicity.[35] All animals dying during the study should be examined at autopsy, even if post-mortem changes are advanced, to attempt to determine the cause of death. Microscopic studies may be done if post-mortem changes permit. It is advisable to kill an animal for pathology studies if it is near death. All animals killed during the study and at termination should be examined at autopsy to detect tumors and gross changes. The autopsies should be complete. All tumors and lesions of uncertain diagnosis by gross examination should be examined microscopically. Although the necessity of examining all tissues in all animals is debatable, since extensive pathology studies would have been done during the toxicity studies, it is advisable to do complete histomorphologic studies on a representative number of high-dose and control animals. If these microscopic studies reveal significant tumors or other changes, then that "target" tissue or organ should be examined microscopically in all animals.

INTERPRETATION OF RESULTS

In addition to anatomical changes due to old age, which sometimes make evaluation of safety by the pathologist difficult, the many types of spontaneous tumors occurring in rodents[7,12,32] create problems of interpretation for both the pathologist and the statistician. A survey of 1,362 CRCD control rats, used during the past 10 years in our laboratory in 12 studies of 56 to 104 weeks' duration, revealed 64 tumors in 26 different organs (Table 4). The frequency of the various tumors ranged from 1 (0.07%) to as many as 210 (15.4%). The most frequently involved organs were the pituitary gland and the mammary gland (Table 5). The incidence of these tumors can vary considerably between groups of control animals. Mammary-tumor incidence from 6% to 52% has been reported for one strain of rat.[28]

In some cases in our studies the less common tumors were seen only in the control animals and not in the approximately 3,000 treated animals (Table 6). If these low-incidence tumors had been found only in the treated group in one of the studies, it is possible that the drug could have been erroneously called a carcinogen by some individuals. Of course, this would not be a statistically valid conclusion. A chemical compound should not be labeled as a carcinogen unless there is a statistically significant increase of the tumor suspected of being induced by that chemical in treated animals over control animals and, preferably, unless there is either a demonstration of a dose-response relation or a consistent increase in all treated groups.

In a recent 96-week study (Table 7) in which

TABLE 4

Spontaneous Tumors in 1,362 Control CRCD Male and Female Rats in 12 Studies (57 to 104 weeks' Duration)

Tissue	Tumors
Adrenal	Adenoma, adenocarcinoma, pheochromocytoma
Brain	Astrocytoma, glioma, neurofibrosarcoma
Cervix	Fibroma
Hematopoietic	Hemangiosarcoma, leukemia
Liver	Adenoma
Lung	Lymphosarcoma, non-chromaffin paraganglioma
Kidney	Carcinoma, cortical adenoma
Mammary gland	Adenoma, fibroadenoma, fibroma, adenocarcinoma, cyst adenoma, papillary-cyst adenoma, papillary-cyst adenocarcinoma
Ovary	Granulosa-cell tumor, papillary-cyst adenocarcinoma
Pancreas	Adenoma, islet-cell carcinoma, acinar-cell adenoma
Parathyroid	Adenoma, adenocarcinoma
Pituitary	Adenoma, adenocarcinoma
Salivary gland	Adenocarcinoma
Sebaceous gland	Carcinoma
Skeleton	Osteogenic sarcoma
Skin	Papilloma, carcinoma, squamous-cell carcinoma, trichoepithelioma, basal-cell carcinoma, fibroadenoma, keratoacanthoma
Spleen	Lymphoma
Striated muscle	Fibrosarcoma, fibroma
Stomach	Papilloma
Testes	Interstitial-cell tumor
Thymus	Carcinoma, sarcoma, thymoma
Thyroid	Adenoma, adenocarcinoma
Urinary bladder	Transitional-cell carcinoma
Uterus	Sarcoma, adenocarcinoma, polyp
Vagina	Leiomyosarcoma
Miscellaneous	Reticulum-cell sarcoma, fibrosarcoma, lipoma, odontoma, liposarcoma, lymphoma, fibroma, sarcoma, lymphosarcoma

TABLE 5

Tumors Found Frequently in 1,362 Control CRCD Male and Female Rats in 12
Studies (57 weeks to 104 weeks' Duration)

Tumor	Number of rats with tumor	%
Mammary adenoma and fibroadenoma	97	7.2
Mammary adenocarcinoma	34	2.5
Pituitary adenoma	210	15.4
Uterine polyp	16	1.2
Fibrosarcoma	9	0.7

TABLE 6

Tumors Found Five Times or Less in 1,222 Control CRCD Male and Female Rats
from 11 Studies (57 to 104 weeks' Duration)

	Number of studies with tumors	
Tumor	In control rats*	Not in treated rats
Adrenal adenoma	3 (5)	—
Adrenal adenocarcinoma	1	—
Adrenal pheochromocytoma	1	—
Astrocytoma	2	1
Glioma	1	1
Neurofibrosarcoma	2	2
Renal carcinoma	2	1
Renal cortical adenoma	1	1
Hemangiosarcoma	1	1
Liposarcoma	1	—
Hepatic adenoma	1	—
Lung lymphosarcoma	1	1
Lymphoma	2 (5)	—
Pancreatic adenosarcoma	1	1
Pancreatic-islet-cell carcinoma	1	—
Sarcoma	3	1
Salivary-gland adenocarcinoma	1	1
Sebaceous-gland carcinoma	1	1
Skin papilloma	1	—
Skin carcinoma	2 (3)	1
Squamous-cell carcinoma	2	1
Trichoepithelioma	1	1
Odontoma	1	1
Osteogenic sarcoma	1	1
Gastric papilloma	2	2
Thymic carcinoma	2 (3)	2
Thymic sarcoma	1	1
Uterine sarcoma	2	1
Uterine adenocarcinoma	1	—
Vaginal leiomyosarcoma	1	1
Cervical fibroma	1	1
Pituitary carcinoma	2 (3)	2
Keratocanthoma	1	1
Urinary-bladder transitional-cell carcinoma	1	1

*Numbers in parentheses indicate the number of rats with tumors.

TABLE 7

Spontaneous Tumors in Control CRCD Rats in a 96-week Study

	Control I		Control II	
Sex	F	M	F	M
Number of rats examined	70	69	69	69
Organ/tumor				
Lung				
non-chromaffin paraganglioma	0	0	1	0
Liver				
hepatocellular adenoma	1	2	1	1
reticulum sarcoma	0	0	1*	0
Kidney				
adenoma	0	1	0	0
Urinary bladder				
transitional-cell carcinoma	1*	0	0	0
Skin				
adenoma	0	0	1	0
lipoma	0	1	0	0
keratoacanthoma	0	1	0	0
squamous-cell carcinoma	0	0	0	1*
basal-cell carcinoma	0	0	0	1
fibroadenoma	0	0	1*	0
Mammary gland				
adenoma	6	0	6	0
fibroadenoma	11	1	11	0
cyst adenoma	–	–	1	–
papillary-cyst adenoma	2	0	2	0
adenocarcinoma	4	0	3	0
papillary-cyst adenocarcinoma	5	0	2	0
Uterus				
polyp	2	–	3	–
Ovary				
granulosa-cell tumor	1*	–	1*	–
papillary-cyst adenocarcinoma	–	–	1*	–
Testes				
interstitial-cell tumor	–	1	–	1
Pituitary				
adenoma	23	14	23	11
adenocarcinoma	5	4	5	2
Adrenal				
pheochromocytoma	1	14	5	4
cortical adenoma	1	2	4	1
Thyroid				
adenoma	1	0	1	1
adenocarcinoma	0	1*	0	0
Pancreas				
islet-cell adenoma	2	4	0	3
acinar-cell adenoma	0	0	0	1
Thymus				
thymoma	0	1	1	1
Spleen				
lymphoma	1	0	0	1
reticulum-cell sarcoma	0	0	0	1*
Brain				
glioma	1*	0	0	0

TABLE 7 (Continued)

	Control I		Control II	
Sex	F	M	F	M
Skeletal Muscle				
fibrosarcoma	0	0	0	2*
Bone				
osteosarcoma	0	1	0	0
myelogenous leukemia	1	0	1	1

*Found only in control animals.

TABLE 8

Differences in Tumor Incidence between Control Groups of CRCD Rats

Date started	Duration (weeks)	Number of rats M	Number of rats F	Tumor Incidence
				Mammary adenocarcinoma
Aug. 1964	77	–	50	12%
Oct. 1964	77	25	25	0
				Pituitary adenoma
Feb. 1967	81	36	36	7%
May 1967	81	15	15	40%
Oct. 1967	81	15	15	12%
Concurrent controls				Pituitary adenoma
I. Nov. 1970	67	80	80	17%
II. Nov. 1970	67	80	80	11%
				Pheochromocytoma
				M F
I. Oct. 1970	96	69	70	20% 1%
II. Oct. 1970	96	69	69	6% 9%

two control groups of 70 male and 70 female rats each were used, 36 tumors were found in 18 different organs and tissues. This is a large variety of tumors in just one study, and of interest is the high frequency of microscopic pheochromocytomas detected by examination of both adrenals of all animals. In this same study, ten types of tumors found in control rats were not found in the 420 treated animals started in the study.

The variation of incidence of specific tumors can be appreciable without apparent relationship to year of birth of the animals (Table 8). This variation can be of importance in evaluating experimental results. In the case of the pheochro-

mocytomas in the rats started in an experiment in October, 1970, Group I males had a high incidence and Group II males had a much lower incidence. The treated males had an incidence of pheochromocytomas similar to that of the Group I rats. If only Group II control rats had been used, it would have been difficult to determine that the higher incidence in the treated group of male rats was not due to treatment.

The demonstration of induced tumors in one species and not in another may suggest metabolic differences in relation to certain compounds. Griseofulvin is a good example of such a compound. During administration of griseofulvin the mouse developed liver tumors, but other species did not. In the mouse the tumor development was due to the formation of hepatic porphyrins. Alteration of porphyrin metabolism was not demonstrated in the rat, guinea pig, or rabbit, and there have been no reports of tumorigenic activity in man.[2,11,17]

POSITIVE CONTROLS

The administration of a known carcinogenic agent to a group of "positive control" animals has been recommended as a part of the routine carcinogenic experiments. The stated purpose of the positive control group is to insure that the animals being used have not lost their sensitivity to carcinogenic agents because of a genetic change. However, this procedure would show only that the animals were sensitive to the carcinogenic agent being given, and that the response was or was not similar to that seen in past experiments. The use of historical background data on the animals being used has not been considered valid by some oncologists and statisticians, since there may have been a genetic change that may have altered the response of the animal to carcinogens. One may ask: If a relatively minor gentic change in the rodent is so important, how can the rodent be used for a determination of the carcinogenic risk for man when the genetic difference is even greater?

A specific carcinogenic agent may induce one or more types of tumors. Another carcinogenic agent may induce different tumors. Also, the tumors induced by a specific carcinogen may vary from none to one or several in different strains of the same species of animals, as well as between different species.[10] Hydrazine sulfate, for example, was reported by Toth to induce tumors in outbred Swiss and inbred C3H mice, but not in inbred AKR mice.[30] Since a drug will usually have a chemical structure different from that of known carcinogens, there is no assurance that the carcinogen selected for the positive control group will predict the sensitivity of the strain or species of animals to the carcinogenic effects of the new drug with unknown activity.[8] It is entirely possible that the strain of animal sensitive to the known carcinogen might be resistant to the carcinogenic effects of the new chemical. A positive control group is useful when the chemical being studied has a structure similar to that of a known carcinogen.[34,35] It is difficult to justify its use as a general procedure for drugs or other chemicals that are not related to a known carcinogen.

Aside from the scientific question of the utility of a positive control group, there are practical considerations. Toxicologists are reluctant to introduce potent known carcinogens or infectious agents into the toxicology laboratory for extended periods of time. There is always a possibility of a breakdown of protective barriers with consequent contamination of animals in other areas of the laboratory. In addition, it is unreasonable to expose laboratory workers for a long period of time to known carcinogens unless absolutely necessary, and then only under extraordinary safety precautions.[34]

The State of Pennsylvania has listed ten dangerous compounds (carcinogens) that cannot be used in industry or research laboratories without special permission and adequate medical surveillance, unless the substances concerned contain 1% or less of a carcinogen.[36] The Department of Labor of the United States was requested by one of the unions and by a consumer group to prohibit exposure of man to ten known carcinogens under threat of court action[37] and has issued emergency safety standards designed to protect workers from harmful exposure to 14 cancer-producing materials used in industry.[38] It is interesting to note that substances containing less than 1% of the carcinogen do not fall within the scope of these restrictions. It is hoped that such regulations will not inhibit cancer research.

The routine incorporation of positive control groups in carcinogenic studies should not be required in view of the questionable value of the procedure and the unnecessary exposure of scientists and animals in laboratories not dedicated to the study of carcinogens. The same philosophy applies to the introduction of pathogenic organisms into a toxicology laboratory. The use of positive control groups can be justified only when a new chemical is structurally similar to a known carcinogen.

A question can arise concerning the situation in which a new chemical or drug is found to be a carcinogen in the animal studies. This is a risk that must be accepted if progress is to be made. Fortunately, according to the oncologists, and as experience has shown, very few classes of chemicals are potent carcinogens.[27]

DISCUSSION

It is obvious that, no matter how much testing is done in animals, there is always the possibility that a drug or other chemical with some carcinogenic activity will not be detected. It is probable, however, that the carcinogenic activity of such agents would be very weak and therefore not present a significant, if any, hazard. In spite of the reluctance of the oncologists to accept the concept of a "no effect" level for carcinogenicity, there may be an exposure level at which the body is able to cope with such agents without detrimental effects,[31] but, unfortunately, it is not possible to prove or disprove this. There has also been a reluctance on the part of some individuals to accept a "no effect" level concept with respect to the toxic effects of drugs. However, it is now recognized that relatively small amounts of drugs can be handled by the body without difficulty.

As stated by Eckhardt,[9] "Materials that produce a profusion of tumors in a variety of species, such as 2-acetylaminofluorene, must be evaluated differently from materials which produce only an occasional tumor in one or two species. In other words, the total available animal data must be carefully evaluated in terms of significance including technicological contribution, and not simply listed or enumerated."

Probably the greatest problem is the interpretation of results of carcinogenic studies where there is no clear indication of enhanced tumor development. The large variety of spontaneous tumors found in very low to relatively high incidence in rodents, and probably in other species of animals as they reach the end of their life span, creates serious problems of statistical and pathological evaluation. There must be clear evidence of a dose–response relation if the range of dosages is adequate, and the incidence of tumors in the control animals must agree with the experience in other studies. The statistician may conclude that there is no significant difference between the treated and control animals, but the pathologist may disagree because a particular tumor has not been observed in the particular species or strain of animal in his experience or reported in the literature. If the tumor incidence in the control group was unusually low, the pathologist may again disagree with the findings of a statistical difference because his historical experience with the varying incidence of tumors among control groups of animals indicated that the low incidence in the control group was by chance and, therefore, the statistical difference was not biologically valid. "An overdependence on statistics can produce fresh difficulties — there is probably no statistic which cannot under some circumstances be misleading."[19] The final interpretation must be based on both biological and statistical evaluations.

In both man and animal there is a latent period from the initiation of exposure to the appearance of an induced tumor that is dose-dependent. This dose–duration relationship should be considered in any decision to use a drug that is potentially carcinogenic but also life-saving or highly effective as a therapeutic agent for a serious disease. For less serious diseases such a drug could be acceptable for treatment of the elderly, who have a relatively short remaining life span, but not for treatment of young or middle-aged individuals, where the potential risk based on the remaining life span would outweigh the potential benefit. It is interesting to note that the latent period in man and animal covers a similar proportion of the total life span of each species.[3]

As stated by Clayson,[6] "No thinking person would wish even one unnecessary carcinogen to be introduced, but the over-rigid exclusion of potential carcinogens may lead to more human suffering than it alleviates." Accordingly, it would be inappropriate to have a strict regulation, such as the Delaney clause, which would forbid the use of agents that have been labeled as potential carcinogens on the basis of animal studies without serious consideration of the benefits that might be derived from such agents. The key word in this statement is "potential" and the basis for using this word must be considered. This adjective is often used following studies of chemicals that show, at best, only questionable carcinogenic activity in animals, or activity in only one strain of a species, in only one species, or activity without consideration of the mechanisms involved. It is not proper to label a chemical as a carcinogen if it is administered in such large doses that the excreted material in the urine exceeds its solubility, resulting in the formation of calculi and the induction of tumors due to irritation.

To label a drug as a carcinogen with potential risk for man because of a slight, and possibly questionable, increase in tumors in animals following life-time administration seems illogical if man does not have life-time exposure. Is it wise to forbid the use of valuable chemicals that in life-time animals studies, using large doses, appear to cause a very low increase of tumors in animals? Since it is difficult, if not impossible, to show lack of carcinogenicity of such agents in man, the easiest decision would be to prohibit exposure of man to such chemicals. Carried to the extreme, no new drug or chemical could ever be classed as a non-carcinogen until all possible experimental procedures have been used to show absence of carcinogenic effects in animals. Even then, by the present trend of extreme conservative thinking, the lack of carcinogenic potential could not be proven.

SUMMARY

At the present time, the only acceptable tests for showing absence of carcinogenic properties of drugs are the 18-month studies in mice and the 24-month studies in rats.

Short-term carcinogenic tests should be accepted for showing lack of carcinogenicity as soon as their validity is demonstrated.

The reason for species-specificity for carcinogenic effects of a chemical should be investigated and evaluated before a chemical is rejected for use.

Agents that are weakly carcinogenic for animals, that is, those that require life-time exposure of large amounts of the chemical in animals for demonstration of activity, probably carry little or no hazard for man, since the latent period in man and animal is proportional to the life span of each. Also, since the carcinogenic effects are related to accumulative exposure, the total human exposure would be much lower than that occurring in animal studies, where large exposure levels are used for the "life span" of the animals.

Proof of carcinogenicity in animals should be unequivocal before the label of "carcinogen" is applied to a chemical.

REFERENCES

1. **Alcock, S. J. and Bond, P. A.,** Observations on the toxicity of Alderlin (pronethalol) in laboratory animals, in *Proc. European Society for the Study of Drug Toxicity,* Vol. 4, Some Factors Affecting Drug Toxicity, International Congress Series No. 81, Excerpta Medica Foundation, Princeton, N.J., 1964, 30.
2. **de C. Baker, S. B. and Davey, D. G.,** The predictive value for man of toxicological tests of drugs in laboratory animals, *Br. Med. Bull.,* 26, 208, 1970.
3. **Boyland, E.,** The biological examination of carcinogenic substances, *Br. Med. Bull.,* 14, 93, 1958.
4. **Boyland, E.,** Carcinogenicity, in *Modern Trends in Toxicology,* Boyland, E. and Goulding, R., Eds., Butterworths, London, 1968, 107.
5. **Clayson, D. B., Lawson, T. A., Santana, S., and Bonser, G. M.,** Correlation between the chemical induction of hyperplasia and of malignancy in the bladder epithelium, *Br. J. Cancer,* 19, 297, 1965.
6. **Clayson, D. B.,** Carcinogenic hazards due to drugs, in *Drug-Induced Diseases,* Vol. 4, Meyler, L. and Peck, H. M., Eds., Excerpta Medica Foundation, Princeton, N.J., 1972, 91.
7. **Crain, R. C.,** Spontaneous tumors in the Rochester strain of the Wistar rat, *Am. J. Pathol.,* 34, 311, 1958.
8. **Della Porta, G.,** The study of chemical substances for possible carcinogenic action. Evaluation of the potential carcinogenic action of a drug, in *Proc. European Society for the Study of Drug Toxicity,* Vol. 3, International Congress Series No. 75, Excerpta Medica Foundation, Princeton, N.J., 1964, 29.
9. **Eckardt, R. E.,** Environmental carcinogenesis: Guest editorial, *Cancer Res.,* 22, 395, 1962.

10. Engbaek, H. C., Bentzon, M. W., Heegaard, H., and Christensen, O., Has isonicotinic acid hydrazide (INH) an oncogenic effect? *Acta Pathol. Microbiol. Scand.*, 65, 69, 1965.

11. Epstein, S., Andrea, J., Joshi, S., and Mantel, N., Hepatocarcinogenicity of griseofulvin following parenteral administration to infant mice, *Cancer Res.*, 27, (Part 1), 1900, 1967.

12. Gilbert, C. and Gillman, J., Spontaneous neoplasms in the albino rat, *S. Afr. J. Med. Sci.*, 23, 257, 1958.

13. Grasso, P. and Golberg, L., Subcutaneous sarcoma as an index of carcinogenic potency, *Food Cosmet. Toxicol.*, 4, 297, 1966.

14. Grasso, P. and Crampton, R. F., The value of the mouse in carcinogenicity testing, *Food Cosmet. Toxicol.*, 10, 418, 1972.

15. Grasso, P., The range of carcinogenic substances in human foods and the problems of testing for them, *Proc. R Soc. Med.*, 66, 26, 1973.

16. Hueper, W. C., Public health hazards from environmental chemical carcinogens, mutagens and teratogens, *Health Phys.*, 21, 689, 1971.

17. Hurst, E. W. and Paget, G. E., Protoporphyrin, cirrhosis and hepatomata in the livers of mice given griseofulvin, *Br. J. Dermatol.*, 75, 105, 1963.

18. Mantel, N. and Bryan, W. R., "Safety" testing of carcinogenic agents, *J. Natl. Cancer Inst.*, 27, 455, 1961.

19. Mantel, N., Some statistical viewpoints in the study of carcinogenesis, in *Progress in Experimental Tumor Research*, Vol. 11, Homburger, F., Ed., S. Karger, Basel/New York, 1967, 431.

20. Mori, K., Yasuno, A., and Matsumoto, K., Induction of pulmonary tumors in mice with isonicotinic acid hydrazid, *Gann*, 51, 83, 1960.

21. Nelson, L. W. and Kelly, W. A., Mesovarial leiomyomas in rats in a chronic toxicity study of soterenol hydrochloride, *Vet. Pathol.*, 8, 452, 1971.

22. Nelson, L. W., Kelly, W. A., and Weikel, J. H., Jr., Mesovarial leiomyomas in rats in a chronic toxicity study of mesuprine hydrochloride, *Toxicol. Appl. Pharmacol.*, 23, 731, 1972.

23. Peacock, P. M., A short term test for carcinogenicity. The effects of certain closely-related polycyclic aromatic hydrocarbons on embryo tissue homografts in BALB/c strain mice, *Br. J. Cancer*, 16, 701, 1962.

24. Peacock, P. M. and Dick, E., A short term test for carcinogenicity. Mouse embryo tissue homografts in BALB/c strain mice, *Br. J. Cancer*, 17, 54, 1963.

25. Rice, J. M., Subcutaneous injections of vaccine adjuvant DEAE-dextran induce local sarcomas in mice, *Nat. New Biol.*, 236, 28, 1972.

26. Rosen, H., Blumenthal, A., Beckfield, W., and Agersborg, H., Jr., Toxicity of a hypoglycemic agent, 2-*p*-methoxy-benzene-sulfonamido-5-isobutyl-1,3,4-thiadiazole, *Toxicol. Appl. Pharmacol.*, 8, 13, 1966.

27. Saffiotti, U., Statement before the Subcommittee on Executive Reorganization and Government Research, Senate Committee on Government Operations, April 7, 1971.

28. Sher, S. P., Mammary tumors in control rats: Literature tabulation, *Toxicol. Appl. Pharmacol.*, 22, 562, 1972.

29. Toth, B., 1,1-Dimethylhydrazine (unsymmetrical) carcinogenesis in mice. Light microscopic and ultrastructural studies on neoplastic blood vessels, *J. Natl. Cancer Inst.*, 50, 181, 1973.

30. Toth, B., Lung tumor induction and inhibition of breast adenocarcinomas by hydrazine sulfate in mice, *J. Natl. Cancer Inst.*, 42, 469, 1969.

31. Weil, C. S., Statistics vs. safety factors and scientific judgment in the evaluation of safety for man, *Toxicol. Appl. Pharmacol.*, 21, 454, 1972.

32. Weisburger, J. H. and Weisburger, E. K., Tests for chemical carcinogens, in *Methods in Cancer Research*, Vol. 1, Busch, H., Ed., Academic Press, New York/London, 1967, 307.

33. Food Protection Committee/Food and Nutrition Board, December 1959, *Problems in the Evaluation of Carcinogenic Hazard from Use of Food Additives*, Publication 749, National Academy of Sciences, National Research Council, Washington, D.C., 1960.

34. FDA Advisory Committee on Protocols for Safety Evaluation (report), Food and Drug Administration Advisory Committee on Protocols for Safety Evaluation: Panel on Carcinogenesis Report on Cancer Testing in the Safety Evaluation of Food Additives and Pesticides, *Toxicol. Appl. Pharmacol.*, 20, 419, 1971.

35. Principles for the Testing and Evaluation of Drugs for Carcinogenicity, Report of a WHO Scientific Group, World Health Organization, Technical Report Series No. 426, Geneva, 1969.

36. Title 25, Rules and Regulations, Part 1, Department of Environmental Resources, Subpart D, Environmental Health and Safety, Article IV, Occupational Health and Safety, Chapter 205 adopted Oct. 14, 1971, Pennsylvania Department of Environmental Resources, Harrisburg, Pa.

37. Nader Group Joins Union in Asking Ban on Ten On-the-job Carcinogens, *Med. World News*, 14, No. 45, 1973.

   Group of Scientists Warns against Ending Ban on Cancer-causing Food Additives, *The New York Times*, January 21, 1973.

38. Emergency Temporary Standard on Certain Carcinogens, *Fed. Register*, 38(5), 10929, 1973.

SECTION 2
REPORT OF DISCUSSION GROUP NO. 1
SPECIES AND STRAIN SELECTION

Michael B. Shimkin

1. For in vivo testing, the species and strains selected should be

a —   available;

b —   economical;

c —   sensitive to carcinogenesis;

d —   stable as to response;

e —   similar to man in regard to metabolism;

f —   similar to man in regard to pathology responses.

2. There is no single bioassay system that is applicable to all compounds or situations, and any present choice is based on empirical experience that must be modified by accruing experience. At the present time, at least two species are necessary for initial evaluation of carcinogenic potential, using both sexes of each species.

3. Genetic stability is as important as a knowledge of the spectrum of spontaneous diseases to which the animals are subject. Inbred strains of mice represent the best available single animal material. They are stable, reproducible, with acceptable background noise, convenient, small, and short-lived. There exists a vast amount of experience with these strains. A wide spectrum of choices within the strains is available, such as:

a —   strain A, for lung, skin, breast tumors

b —   strain C_3H for subcutaneous breast and liver tumors

c —   strain BALB/c for lung, skin lymphoma

d —   strain C57Bk, for lymphoma

e — F_1 hybrids, CxA, C57xC_3H, etc.

4. The rat is also a desirable species. It is easy to breed, has few serious diseases, is of convenient size, usually docile, and is economical to house. There is a large volume of information on rats, including incidence of spontaneous tumors and response to known carcinogens. Rats are especially sensitive to aromatic amines, azo-compounds, and radiation. The Sprague-Dawley strain has a relatively high incidence of mammary tumors and the Fischer 344 strain has a high incidence of testicular tumors, whereas the AXC rats have low occurrence of tumors. In general, spontaneous malignant tumors are rare in rats.

5. Inbred Syrian hamsters are probably the next-best species, but experience with them is still limited. They have a low tumor-background incidence.

6. Larger species, including primates, are impractical for bioassays, and they should be restricted to special problems. Further exploration of additional species, particularly non-rodents, is desirable.

7. The sources of animals must be limited to those following standard requirements for animal breeding and having periodic re-accreditations, such as those of A.A.A.L.A.C.

8. All animals must be healthy and must be *maintained* on standard diets and in standard environments. They must be defined in regard to their infectious disease spectrum as far as possible.

9. In all tests, and with all species and strains, appropriate parallel controls are essential.

SECTION 3

REPORT OF DISCUSSION GROUP NO. 2
DIETS

Paul M. Newberne

Components of diet can alter markedly the progress of chemical carcinogenesis in rodents and probably in other animals as well. A classical example, and one of the few that is understood, is the enhancement of DAB carcinogenesis by riboflavin deficiency, in which deficient hepatic metabolism of DAB is depressed.[1] Less specific is the general depression of tumor induction and growth in animals fed insufficient calories.[2] In designing diets to be fed to animals in which the carcinogenic potential of drugs is to be determined, certain questions must be asked and then answered as completely as possible from a review of published work and of experiments in progress. This process will lead to recommendations for diets to be used and also point to areas in which further work is needed. Questions to be discussed, and partial answers available at present, are as follows:

1. In testing chemicals for carcinogenicity in rodents, do we want to use diets to maximize the animals' response, to mimic human diet, and/or to standardize the conditions of the animal from one experiment to another?

The safety of people exposed to the chemicals requires that testing be done in animals and under conditions in which the greatest likelihood exists that potential human carcinogens will be detected. A second requirement is that standardization of animals and technique be achieved insofar as is practically possible in order that experiments can be repeated and results from different laboratories compared. Attempts to mimic human diets would be premature at present, except for examining specific conditions and chemicals indicated by epidemiologic studies, such as those reviewed recently by Shils.[3]

2. Are there generalizations that can be made about effects of diet on experimental chemical carcinogenesis that can be used to design an experimental diet?

There is evidence from several laboratories that chow diets or other diets composed of unrefined natural ingredients decrease tumor yield in rats given chemical or hormonal carcinogens and in X-irradiated mice, compared to tumor yield in animals fed semisynthetic purified diets.[a,b] This may be the result of induction of drug-metabolizing enzymes (DME) in liver, intestine and lung by vegetable components or insecticides or other contaminants of the chow diets, or of variable drug-metabolizing enzyme levels due to nutrient variation in chow (Table 1). The induction of drug-metabolizing enzymes has been shown generally to decrease carcinogenesis by several different chemicals[c] (Table 2).

Dietary protein levels have not affected carcinogenesis consistently within the range of protein that supports adequate growth. Severe protein deficiency retards tumor growth and depresses hepatic drug-metabolizing enzymes.[d]

Dietary fat does not affect tumor development consistently. Lipotropic nutrients (choline, methionine, folic acid, and vitamin B_{12}) have been found to influence both toxicity and carcinogenicity of chemicals, although not always in a consistent pattern. Early studies implicated deficiency of these nutrients in enhancement of the induction of hepatocarcinomas by what we now know to be aflatoxin, but others suggested an inhibition of DAB carcinogenesis by vitamin B_{12} deficiency.[4,5] Recent studies have shown that deficiency of lipotropes decreases the acute toxicity of both the pyrrolizidine alkaloids and aflatoxin B_1 (AFB_1) but enhances the chronic

---

[a]Chow diets protected female rats against 2-acetylaminofluorene (2-AAF)-induced hepatic, mammary and bladder tumors, compared to a defined stock diet.[24]

[b]Natural-product diets protected female rats against 2-AAF-induced mammary and ear-duct tumors, compared to semisynthetic diet.[12]

[c]Chow-fed female rats had greater basal levels of aryl hydrocarbon hydroxylase activity in liver, lung, and small intestine than rats fed semisynthetic diet.[19,20]

[d]Protein, hepatic N-demethylase, and aryl hydrocarbon hydroxylase correlated positively with dietary casein level.[15a]

TABLE 1

Nutrient Variations in Chow Diets

Ingredient	NAS requirements	Amounts found in chows* by laboratory analysis
Calcium, %	0.56	(0.5, 0.27, 0.89) (0.95, 0.41, 0.82) (1.4, 0.72)
Copper, mg/kg – ppm	5.6	(3.8, 6.9, 65) (19.7, 39.0, 90) (3.2, 6.0, 76.0)
Iodine, mg/kg – ppm	0.17	(0.10, 0.96) (1.78, 0.23) (0.09, 1.23, 2.0)
Zinc, mg/kg – ppm	13.3	(20, 17, 10) (16.3, 5.0) (38.4, 9.1)
Vitamin D, IU/kg	1,111	(987, 1,264, 4,100) (2,958, 1,023, 2,847) (3,684, 620, 5,450)
Vitamin A, mg retinyl/kg	0.67	(0.28, 0.77, 0.57) (1.96, 0.55, 0.13) (0.20, 0.65) (1.49, 0.16)
Riboflavin, mg/kg – ppm	2.8	(5.7, 2.1. 8.9) (0.9, 38.4) (3.2, 1.0, 5.9)
Vitamin B_{12}, mg/kg – ppm	0.0056	(0.0023, 0.0097) (0.0011, 0.0075) (0.0011, 0.0027) (0.0019, 0.0095)
DDT, ppm	–	(0, 17) (5, 0, 27)
Nitrates, ppm	–	(20, 0, 200) (6, 90)

*Each set of data enclosed in parentheses represents a different brand.

toxicity and carcinogenicity of AFB_1 (Table 3). The same deficiency enhances nitrosamine carcinogenesis. The deficiency may affect the action of chemicals by its depression of hepatic drug metabolism. Biochemical interactions between nitrosamine and hepatic lipotrope stores and the enzymes related to them have been demonstrated.[6]

Specific effects of some vitamins and minerals have been demonstrated with specific carcinogens, e.g., deficiency of vitamin A enhanced colon carcinogenesis by AFB_1 but not by dimethyl-hydrazine.[7,8] As with dietary protein and lipid, no consistent effect on tumor induction or development has been found within the range of vitamin and mineral levels sufficient to maintain growth.

3. By what mechanisms may diet affect chemical carcinogenesis?

Examples of dietary effects on drug metabolism and carcinogenesis have been given above. Two

TABLE 2

Inhibition of Carcinogenesis by Induction of Increased Microsomal Enzyme Activity

Carcinogen	Inducer	Species	Organ	References
3'-Methyl-4-dimethyl-aminoazobenzene	Polycyclic hydrocarbons	Rat	Liver	16, 17 30
Urethane	β-Naphthoflavone, Chlordane, phenobarbital	Mouse	Lung	24
7,12-Dimethylbenz (a)-anthracene	Polycyclic hydrocarbons	Rat	Breast	15, 22
7,12-Dimethylbenz (a)-anthracene	β-Naphthoflavone	Mouse	Lung	21

TABLE 3

Effect of Experimental Diets on Hepatic Drug-metabolizing Enzymes[18]

Diet[a]	Number of rats[b]	Aminopyrine demethylase[c]	p-Nitroanisole demethylase[c]	Benzpyrene hydroxylase[c]
1	12	481 ± 55	1,132 ± 74	184 ± 16
2	12	305 ± 23	536 ± 116	99 ±11
p value[d]		<0.05	<0.01	<0.01

[a]Diet 1, adequate; diet 2, marginally lipotrope-deficient.
[b]Four rats were used for each enzyme assay, so the total number examined per diet was 12.
[c]Enzymes were measured in liver homogenate and expressed per gram of dry, fat-free liver ± SE. Units are aminopyrine demethylase, μg aminoantipyrine/hr; p-nitroanisole demethylase, μg p-nitrophenol/hr; benzpyrene hydroxylase, quinine units.[15a]
[d]Calculated from Student t test using two-sided probability for diet 1 vs. diet 2.

other possible mechanisms of dietary action are through changes in intestinal flora and in immunological processes.

There is epidemiologic and bacteriologic evidence of a relationship between diet, intestinal bacteria, and carcinoma of colon and breast.[9,10] The relationship is thought to be mediated through bacterial metabolism of either endogenous or exogenous carcinogens present in intestinal contents.

Immunologic processes important in carcinogenesis are just beginning to be investigated. Deficits in cell-mediated immunity resulting in defective surveillance for abnormal cells have been postulated to be a cause of tumor development. Diet affects immunologic processes, and recent studies have shown that protein deficiency and lipotrope deficiency in rats and folic acid deficiency in people suppress cell-mediated immunity. In the rat model, the depression is associated with increased susceptibility to tumor development.[e]

4. Aside from effects on carcinogenesis, what degree of standardization of diets can be achieved?

Chow diets, even from the same manufacturer, vary greatly in their nutrient content and composition and in the extent of chemical contamination. Therefore, uniformity can be assured only within a single lot. Semisynthetic diets composed of refined ingredients have been formulated for laboratory rodents and used extensively.[8] Their use assures

[e]Diet, cell-mediated immunity, and tumor growth: protein deficiency depresses cell-mediated immunity (CMI) and growth of transplanted tumors in mice;[11] lipotrope deficiency or protein deficiency in female rats depresses CMI in offspring;[13] folate deficiency depresses CMI in people.[14]

uniformity of dietary intake and has proved satisfactory in long-term studies. The level of protein in diets currently in use may be too high to sustain normal renal function and probably should be lowered somewhat, but otherwise the diets are satisfactory.

In cases where carcinogenicity of a chemical is suspected but not clearly demonstrated in animals fed a standardized adequate diet, one may wish to repeat the studies using a diet marginally deficient in lipotropes, or perhaps in protein, in an attempt to enhance the sensitivity of the animal to carcinogenesis.

RECOMMENDATIONS

In view of the above considerations, we propose the following recommendations of choice of diet for experimental animals used in testing of drugs for carcinogenesis.

I. STANDARDIZATION-REPRODUCIBILITY

Assured Sensitivity

A. Use semisynthetic diets free of known enzyme inducers and antioxidants.
B. Feed *ad libitum.*

C. Provide adequate, standardized levels and sources of protein, fat, carbohydrates, vitamins, and minerals.

SUBRECOMMENDATIONS FOR FURTHER RESEARCH

We need to specify, insofar as possible, how dietary standardization relates to sensitivity to carcinogenesis. Therefore, we need to define how diet affects carcinogenesis in terms of physiogeochemical mechanisms. In addition to research required to define this relationship, examination of the effects of dietary manipulation on carcinogenesis also may provide important clues on the fundamental carcinogenic mechanism. Therefore, certain fundamental areas of research need to be further investigated.

1. Effects of dietary manipulation on microsomal enzyme activities, and the relationship of these activities to carcinogenicity.
2. Effects of dietary manipulation on cell-mediated immunity and its relationship to carcinogenicity.
3. Effects of dietary manipulation on sensitivity of target tissues to carcinogens.

REFERENCES

1. Kensler, C. J., Sugiura, K., Young, N. F., Halter, C. R., and Rhoads, C. P., *Science,* 93, 308, 1941.
2. Tannenbaum, A., in *Physiopathology of Cancer,* 2nd ed., Homberger, F., Ed., Phiebig, White Plains, N.Y., 1959, 517.
3. Shils, M. E., *CA Cancer J. Clin.,* p. 399, 1971.
4. Day, P. L., Payne, L. D., and Dinning, J. S., *Proc. Soc. Exp. Biol. Med.,* 74, 854, 1950.
5. Miller, E. C., Plescia, A. M., Miller, J. A., and Heidelberger, C., *J. Biol. Chem.,* 196, 863, 1952.
6. Poirier, L. and Whitehead, V. M., *Cancer Res.,* 33, 383, 1973.
7. Newberne, P. M. and Rogers, A. E., *J. Natl. Cancer Inst.,* 50, 439, 1973.
8. Rogers, A. E., Herndon, B. J., and Newberne, P. M., *Cancer Res.,* 33, 1003, 1973.
9. Burkett, D. P., *Cancer,* 28, 3, 1971.
10. Drasar, B. S. and Irving, D., *Br. J. Cancer,* 27, 167, 1973.
11. Jose, D. G. and Good, R. A., *Cancer Res.,* 33, 807, 1973.
12. Engel, R. W. and Copeland, D. H., *Cancer Res.,* 12(1):211, 1952.
13. Gebhard, B. and Newberne, P. M., *Brit. J. Immunol.,* in press, 1974.
14. Gross, R. L., Reid, J. V. O., Newberne, P. M., Burgess, B., Marston, R., and Hift, W., *Amer. J. Clin. Nutr.,* in press, 1974.
15. Huggins, C., Lorraine, G., and Fukunishi, R., *Proc. Natl. Acad. Sci.,* 51:737, 1964.
15a. McLeon, A. E. M. and McLeon, E. K., *Biochem. J.,* 100:564, 1966.
16. Miller, E. C., Miller, J. A., Brown, R. R., and MacDonald, J. C., *Cancer Res.,* 18:469, 1958.
17. Richardson, H. L., Stein, A. R., and Borson-Nacht-Nebel, E., *Cancer Res.,* 12:356, 1952.
18. Rogers, A. E. and Newberne, P. M., *Toxicol. Appl. Pharmacol.,* 20:113, 1971.
19. Wattenberg, L. W., *Cancer Res.,* 28(1):99, 1971.
20. Wattenberg, L. W., *Toxicol. Appl. Pharmacol.,* 23:741, 1972.
21. Wattenberg, L. W. and Leong, J. L., *Proc. Soc. Exp. Biol. Med.,* 128:940, 1968.
22. Wheatley, D. N., *Brit. J. Cancer,* 22:787, 1968.
23. Wilson, R. H. and DeEds, F., *Arch. Ind. Hyg. Occup. Med.,* 1:73, 1950.
24. Yamamoto, R. S., Weisburger, J. H., and Weisburger, E. K., *Cancer Res.,* 31:483, 1971.

SECTION 4
REPORT OF DISCUSSION GROUP NO. 3
DOSE SELECTION AND ADMINISTRATION

Leo Friedman*

The panel was charged with the responsibility of producing guidelines for the selection of dose levels and routes of administration appropriate for the evaluation of carcinogenic activity of new drugs. In its 8-hour deliberations, the panel identified and considered the various elements of these aspects of the testing protocol and aimed at a series of tentative recommendations.

The panel did not consider the implication of co-carcinogenesis, anti-carcinogenesis, initiation, or promotion as factors influencing the assay of carcinogenic response. In general, these phenomena are poorly understood, and it is impossible to assess their significance in this context.

The essential objective of the carcinogenesis evaluation study is to detect in the most appropriate way available any evidence of carcinogenic potential the substance under study can evoke. This evidence is essential for providing the most complete and reliable background of information against which an accurate risk/benefit analysis may be made. The assay protocol, therefore, should maximize the sensitivity of the test without altering its accuracy. Among all the aspects of carcinogenesis bioassay protocols under study by the various panels, the question of dose and route of administration has the greatest bearing on sensitivity and accuracy. Concern with maximizing the sensitivity of the test has led to the concept of the maximum tolerated dose.

This term has almost as many different connotations as there are individuals who use it. The ambiguities tend to distract attention from the important biological questions inherent in carcinogenesis or mutagenesis bioassay. We propose that a sharper focus on these questions would result from dropping this term. Our concern will be with the selection of the maximum test dose for each carcinogenesis bioassay.

Valid interpretations of results can be vitiated by depressed growth rates, non-specific injury or irritation of target tissues, excessive stimulation of glandular activity through normal mechanisms, and abnormal pharmacological effects of excessive dosage.

*Deceased

With respect to the issue of maximum dose in this frame of reference, it was noted that the objective was to administer the highest possible dose that will permit valid interpretation of the experimental observations. In most tests, the highest dose meets the following criteria:

1. It will not produce depression in weight gain of more than 10%, as compared with the controls, in rodents; nor a difference of 10% in weight of treated and control animals of other species.

2. It will allow at least 50% of the treated animals to survive to the end of the study, provided that intercurrent infections do not reduce viability of the test animals.

3. It will not produce pharmacologic effects that will interfere with completion of the study or otherwise invalidate the result.

At least two lower dose levels should be chosen, the second-highest dose ordinarily being 10 to 50% of the maximum.

During the discussion it became evident that there were two aspects to a carcinogenesis bioassay that would strongly influence dose selection. The first is concerned essentially with the question of whether the drug is a carcinogen or not; the selection of the proper maximum dose is crucial for obtaining a valid answer to this question. The second is concerned with relative carcinogenic potency; there should be enough valid information on this point to enable the most accurate estimation of risk, should the circumstances warrant consideration of the use of this substance because of the benefit to be derived. This aspect would require consideration of what the lowest and intermediate dose levels should be. In most cases the primary, if not the only, concern is with the first question. However, proper consideration of the second question cannot be avoided when the study is designed to provide definitive data on chronic toxicity as well as on carcinogenicity. Otherwise the study is simply a screening test for carcinogenicity and must be followed by another life-time study to properly delineate all aspects of chronic toxicity. In the use of a drug that is negative for carcinogenicity or must be considered for use because of its outstanding beneficial potential, the low dose in a test must in some way approximate the human use level.

Adminsisration of the test substance should begin at conception and continue through the completion of the experiment or death.

FREQUENCY OF DOSING

Under the usual circumstances, the animals should be treated from 5 to 7 days each week until death. In tests designed specifically to evaluate the carcinogencitiy of drugs, it is undesirable to stop dosing before the end of the experiment. Nevertheless, if further studies are necessary to complete the risk/benefit evaluation of a drug, short-term dosing may be appropriate.

ROUTE OF ADMINISTRATION

Many factors determine route of administration, including the proposed route of application of the drug on humans, its phamacokinetic characteristics following various routes of administration, and the effects this will have on the metabolic action and detoxication of the drug. The following precepts may be useful:

1. If the route of human use is oral, exposure of the animals should also be oral, except in circumstances where pharmacokinetic observations suggest the contrary. There is no compelling reason to provide guidelines for choosing between administration of the test material in the drinking water, in the diet, or by gavage. The judgment of the investigators, based on their knowledge of the specific situation, should be determining.

2. If the substance is to be used in man topically, it is suggested that the material should also be applied topically in the animal assay. However, it was noted that present knowledge of skin carcinogenesis in rats and guinea pigs indicates that these species are of little value for detecting skin carcinogenesis. Because of the small amounts of the test compounds that can be applied topically, it is often necessary to use the oral route additionally.

3. Parenteral administration, i.e., intramuscular or subcutaneous injection, should be used only if the test compound is poorly absorbed after administration by the oral route. If such injections must be used in rodents, particularly rats, it is necessary to place more emphasis on the yield of tumors remote from the injection site than on that of tumors occurring locally. In general, parenteral administration must be restricted by the undesirable local effects. In many studies injection once a week has been the maximum frequency the animals will tolerate.

4. The use of inhalation exposure should be limited, because available animal models are not sufficiently established to yield valid negative results with substances of unknown carcinogenic potency. It is preferable to accept negative findings from another route of exposure.

In all tests for carcinogenic acitivity of drugs it is desirable to simulate the expected route of human exposure. For the proper evaluation of these tests, it is essential to avoid creating entirely artificial situations; during parenteral administration, particularly, it may be necessary to use a different vehicle for the test chemical than for the final product. Decisions about the choice of vehicle should be made in light of previous experience of the behavior of substances similar to the test compound and are best left to the judgment of the investigator.

SECTION 5
REPORT OF DISCUSSION GROUP NO. 4
INCEPTION AND DURATION OF TESTS

L. Tomatis

As with other possible environmental hazards to man, an investigation of the possible carcinogenicity of new drugs can be carried out by following one of two approaches: (1) to maximize the sensitivity of bioassay systems regarding potential carcinogenicity of the drug under test by giving it to a susceptible species over a prolonged period of time, including the most sensitive age, or (2) to adopt an experimental testing protocol most similar to human exposure.

The group is in favor of the first approach for the following reasons: (1) drugs are likely to be given to people at a particularly high risk, e.g., pregnant women, children, or patients who may have altered metabolic capacities or impaired immune defences; (2) the exposure levels can be precisely evaluated; (3) since a risk-versus-benefit evaluation has been accepted in the past (e.g., administration of cytostatic drugs to cancer patients), it should be done with full awareness of any possible risk; (4) it is not sure that a drug marketed initially for a specific use will not be used later for different purposes or given to a different category of patients or consumed by the general population through food.

In addition, one also frequently hears the assertion that almost any substance is carcinogenic if enough is administered. The available experimental evidence does not substantiate this notion. Most substances tested by the National Cancer Institute have, in fact, been negative even when given in large doses to immature mice. In particular, only 11 of 120 chemicals that were already selected for their possible carcinogenicity were found definitely carcinogenic in the mouse.[13] Fears that any new drug tested by a sensitive bioassay procedure will prove carcinogenic appear to be without foundation, and the negative results expected from the majority of such tests will be much more reassuring than results obtained from the less sensitive conventional studies in adult animals.

The group has reviewed recommendations made by several committees or learned scholars, in particular for the inception and duration of tests, following up a review by a UICC (International Union Against Cancer) Committee in 1969[2] (see Tables 1 and 2).

There is a definite tendency to consider observation for at least two years as adequate duration of a negative test. This tendency appears to have been constant, apart from a few exceptions, during the last 15 years. For the inception of tests, however, there has been an evident change of attitude in recent years. Following the pioneer experiments of Pietra et al.,[19] neonatal treatment was a great favorite and for a while was claimed as possibly being the most sensitive testing model. Reviews of the available data now indicate that neonatal treatment alone can be recommended in some instances, but cannot be recommended as a general procedure.[5] More recently, following results obtained in experimental transplacental carcinogenesis and in epidemiological studies, prenatal exposure has received much attention, particularly the aspects enumerated below. (1) Prenatal exposure of rats to certain nitrosamides is followed by a high incidence of tumors in the offspring.[6,15] (2) Tumors in the offspring, especially tumors of the CNS and PNS (central and peripheral nervous systems), appear following treatment of pregnant rats at a dose level that does not produce tumors in the mothers.[14,28] (3) Prenatal exposure to a chemical increases the susceptibility of the offspring to the carcinogenic effect of the same chemical or of another chemical later in life; the carcinogenic effect of the chemical is expressed in the same target organ.[18,31,32] (4) When genetically resistant animals are exposed *in utero* to a carcinogen, not only do many more tumors develop than when exposure occurs during adult life,[24] but a high proportion of these grow rapidly and behave as malignant tumors, as in genetically susceptible strains, and are highly antigenic in syngeneic recipients;[25] transplacental exposure, therefore, can circumvent genetically determined resistance. (5) Diethylstilbestrol, a chemical for which carcinogenicity had been

TABLE 1

Comparison of Recommendations of Different Committees

	EUROTOX	FAO/WHO	British Ministry of Health	Food Protection Committee, U.S.A.
Species and route of administration	Rats – feeding Mice – feeding Mice – repeated injection Rats – repeated injection	Rats – feeding Mice – feeding	Rats – feeding Mice – feeding Mice – repeated injection Rats – repeated injection	Rats – feeding Mice – feeding Dogs – feeding Mice – skin application Mice – single injection
Number of animals of each group which should survive	15	20	12	50*
Duration of tests	Rats – 2 years Mice – 80 weeks	Rats – 2 years Mice – 80 weeks	Rats – 2 years Mice – 80 weeks	Rats – life span Mice – life span Dogs – 4 years

*This number is presumably the number of animals at the start of the test.

TABLE 2

Comparison of Recommendations of Different Committees or Learned Scholars

Year	Purpose of testing	Inception of test	Duration of test
1958[1]	General testing	Non specified, but a 3-generation treatment is recommended in some instances	Life span or 2 years for mice, 2½ years for rats
1959[19]	Food additives	Adolescent animals; fetal exposure might be of value in some instances	2 years or more
1961[9]	Food additives	Soon after weaning	Life span
1967[4]	Drugs	Young adults; in some cases neonatal treatment or, preferably, prenatal exposure followed by a few weeks' postnatal exposure	Life span
1967[21]	Drugs	Not specified	Life span
1969[20]	Pesticides	Young animals	Life span (however, 18 months of observation was found adequate in some instances)
1969[2]	General testing	Soon after weaning; in some instances neonatal treatment	Long finite period, or life span
1969[18]	Drugs	Soon after weaning; in some instances neonatal treatment	At least 18 months in mice, or 2 years in rats
1971[3]	General testing	Not specified	Life span
1971[10]	Food additives and pesticides	Prior to conception and continued in the offspring	2 years

demonstrated in five animal species, was shown to be carcinogenic to man following prenatal exposure.[11,12]

So far, tumors of the offspring have been reported in five animal species (mouse, rat, hamster, guinea pig, and pig) following prenatal exposure to at least 30 substances of various chemical structures, such as urethane, polycyclic hydrocarbons, N-nitroso compounds, cycasin, aflatoxin, etc., adminstered by different routes (Table 3).[29]

There seems to be little doubt that some tissues are more susceptible to certain carcinogens during fetal and/or infant life than later on. This is the case, in particular, with nervous tissue and with certain N-nitroso compounds. Unpublished results[17,26] indicate, however, that prenatal exposure of rats to dimethylbenzanthracene (DMBA) is also followed by the occurrence of tumors of the nervous system, which would indicate the general higher susceptibility of fetal nervous tissue, compared to that of adults, to a variety of carcinogens during intrauterine life.

While the chemical structure and route of administration seem irrelevant for the effect revealed by prenatal exposure, the timing of treatment during pregnancy appears to be critical. Exposure during the first half of pregnancy results in an embryotoxic effect and, later, in a teratogenic effect, whereas exposure in the second half of pregnancy results in a carcinogenic effect. A possible explanation for the absence of a carcinogenic effect in early and, in some instances, even in late pregnancy is the lack of adequate metabolic competence of fetal tissues. Metabolic competence is progressively and asynchronously acquired by different fetal tissues during their development, and certain chemicals do not exert a carcinogenic effect in the progeny if the mother is exposed prior to the last few days of pregnancy, as is the case with dimethylnitrosamine (DMN) for instance.[6,16]

TABLE 3

TABLE 3

Chemical Carcinogens Inducing Tumors Following Prenatal Exposure

Urethane	Ethylnitrosourea (and ethylurea + Na nitrite)	1-Methyl-2-benzylhydrazine
o-Aminoazotoluene	Nitrosomethylurea	1-Phenyl-3,3-dimethyltriazene
7,12-Dimethylbenz[a]anthracene	Ethylnitrosobiuret	1-Phenyl-3,3-diethyltriazene
Benzo[a]pyrene	1,2-Diethylhydrazine	1-Pyridyl-3,3-diethyltriazene
Methylcholanthrene	Azoethane	Dimethylsulfate
Crude cycad material (methylazoxymethanol)	Azoxyethane	Diethylsulfate
Diethylnitrosamine	Azoxymethane	
Dimethylnitrosamine	Nitrosomethylurethane	1,3-Propane sultone
Elasiomycin	Ethylnitrosourethane	Methyl methanesulfonate
n-Propylnitrosourea	Aflatoxin B	^{32}P-phosphate
	N-Isopropyl-α-(2-methyl-hydrazino)-p-toluamide, HCl (procarbazine, Natulan)	Stilbestrol

Not only may fetal tissues be insensitive to the carcinogenic effect of a chemical if exposed at too early an age, but the sensitivity of the tissues may change at different stages of development and a carcinogenic effect may be observed in different target organs.[8,15,30] Prenatal exposure to a chemical may result in the appearance of tumors at different sites than in cases where the chemical is given postnatally.[7] A reduction in the tumor-latency period in offspring compared to that of their mothers, which could also be taken as an indication of the higher sensitivity of fetal than of maternal tissues, was observed with some, but not all, carcinogens tested.[29]

In addition, all chemicals that up to now have been proved to result in the occurrence of tumors following their administration to pregnant animals were already known to produce tumors in adult and/or newborn animals. At present we may, therefore, only speculate that prenatal exposure per se would reveal the carcinogenic effect of a chemical that otherwise would not have been revealed by tests carried out in newborn or young-adult animals.

Therefore, although prenatal exposure may reveal a carcinogenic effect at unusual target sites and at very low levels of exposure, it cannot be recommended as a general routine procedure that could per se replace conventional testing on young adults. A more sensitive procedure would be to integrate prenatal exposure with long-term postnatal exposure, in order to maximize the sensitivity of the bioassay system.

The group recommends that the parents should be mated at eight to nine weeks of age (rats and mice) and exposed to the chemical under test during the second half of pregnancy (e.g., day 12 for rats). Their exposure should continue for the desired duration, and they would then constitute a group of young adults under conventional long-term tests. Their offspring, which may have been exposed already in utero and postnatally through the maternal milk and excreta, should then be directly exposed for as long as desired from the time they are weaned. This procedure would result in two different experimental groups, one composed of the parent generation and a second composed of the offspring (F_1).

The group recommends as duration of the test a long finite period, which is more practical than total-life-span studies, because a few animals may far exceed the normal life span of the species and therefore unnecessarily extend the duration of the experiment.

It is recommended that no test be accepted as negative unless a statistically significant proportion of the test animals survive for 24 months in the case of mice, and 30 months in the case of rats. Experience gained in many laboratories has indicated that with proper husbandry a number of strains of mice and rats survive long enough to meet these requirements.

REFERENCES

1.   Boyland, E., The biological examination of carcinogenic substances, *Br. Med. Bull.*, 14, 93, 1958.
2.   Berenblum, I., Ed., *Carcinogenicity Testing*, UICC, Geneva, Switzerland, 1969.
3.   *Chemicals and the Future of Man*, U.S. Government Printing Office, Washington, D.C., 1971, 180.
4.   Della Porta, G., Some aspects of medical drug testing for carcinogenic activity, in *Potential Carcinogenic Hazards from Drugs*, UICC Monographs Ser. 7, Truhaut, R., Ed., Springer-Verlag, New York, 1967, 33.
5.   Della Porta, G. and Terracini, B., Chemical carcinogenesis in infant animals, *Prog. Exp. Tumor Res.*, 11, 334, 1969.
6.   Druckrey, H., Chemical structure and action in transplacental carcinogenesis and teratogenesis, in *Transplacental Carcinogenesis*, Scientific Publication No. 4, Tomatis, L. and Mohr, U., Eds., International Agency for Research on Cancer, Lyon, France, 1973, 45.
7.   Druckrey, H. and Landschutz, C. H., Transplazentare und neonatale Krebserzeugung durch Methylnitrosobiuret (ANBY) an BDIX Ratten, *Z. Krebsforsch.*, 76, 45, 1971.
8.   Druckrey, H., Schagan, B., and Ivankovic, S., Erzeugung neurogener Malignome durch einmalige Gabe von Aethylnitrosoharnstoff (ANH) an neugeborene und junge BDIX Ratten, *Z. Krebsforsch.*, 74, 141, 1970.
9.   Evaluation of the carcinogenic hazards of food additives, *W.H.O. Tech. Rep. Ser.*, No. 220, 1961.
10. Food and Drug Administration Advisory Committee Protocols for Safety Evaluation, Panel on Carcinogenesis Report on Cancer Testing in the Safety Evaluation of Food Additives and Pesticides, *Toxicol. Appl. Pharmacol.*, 20, 419, 1971.
11. Herbst, A. L., Ulfelder, H., and Poskanzer, D. C., Adenocarcinoma of the vagina: Association of maternal stilbestrol therapy with tumor appearance in young women, *N. Engl. J. Med.*, 284, 878, 1971.
12. Herbst, A. L., Kurman, R. J., Scully, R. E., and Poskanzer, D. C., Clear-cell adenocarcinoma of the genital tract in young females. Registry reports, *N. Engl. J. Med.*, 287, 1259, 1972.
13. Innes, J. R. M., Ulland, B. M., Valerio, M. G., Petrucelli, L., Fishbein, L., Hart, E. R., Pallotta, A. J., Bates, R. R., Falk, H. L., Gart, J. J., Klein, M., Mitchell, I., and Peters, J., Bioassay of pesticides and industrial chemicals for tumorigenicity in mice: A preliminary note, *J. Natl. Cancer Inst.*, 42, 1101, 1969.
14. Ivankovic, S., Experimental prenatal carcinogenesis, in *Transplacental Carcinogenesis*, Scientific Publication No. 4, Tomatis, L. and Mohr, U., Eds., International Agency for Research on Cancer, Lyon, France, 1973, 92.
15. Ivankovic, S. and Druckrey, H., Tranzplazentare Erzeugung von malignen Tumoren des Nervensystems. I. Aethylnitrosoharnstoff (ANH) an BDIX Ratten, *Z. Krebsforsch.*, 71, 320, 1968.
16. Magee, P. N., Mechanisms of transplacental carcinogenesis by nitroso compounds, in *Transplacental Carcinogenesis*, Scientific Publication No. 4, Tomatis, L. and Mohr, U., Eds., International Agency for Research on Cancer, Lyon, France, 1973, 143.
17. Napalkov, N. P., personal communication.
18. Napalkov, N. P., Some general considerations on the problem of transplacental carcinogenesis, in *Transplacental Carcinogenesis*, Scientific Publication No. 4, Tomatis, L. and Mohr, U., Eds., International Agency for Research on Cancer, Lyon, France, 1973, 1.
19. Pietra, G., Spencer, K., and Shubik, P., Response of newly born mice to a chemical carcinogen, *Nature*, 183, 1689, 1959.
20. Prevention of cancer, *W.H.O. Tech. Rep. Ser.*, No. 276, 1964.
21. Principles for the testing and evaluation of drugs for carcinogenicity, *W.H.O. Tech. Rep. Ser.*, No. 426, 1969.
22. *Problems in the Evaluation of Carcinogenic Hazard from Use of Food Additives*, NAS-NRC Publication No. 749, National Academy of Sciences, Washington, D.C., 1960.
23. Report of the Secretary's Commission on Pesticides and their Relationship to Environmental Health, U.S. Department of Health, Education and Welfare, Washington, D.C., 1969.
24. Rice, J. M., Transplacental carcinogenesis in mice by 1-ethyl-1-nitrosourea, *Ann. N.Y. Acad. Sci.*, 163, 813, 1969.
25. Rice, J. M., Biological behavior of transplacentally induced tumors in mice, in *Transplacental Carcinogenesis*, Scientific Publication No. 4, Tomatis, L. and Mohr, U., Eds., International Agency for Research on Cancer, Lyon, France, 1973, 71.
26. Rice, J. M., personal communication.
27. Shubik, P., A program for the investigation of the possible chronic hazards of drugs, in *Potential Carcinogenic Hazards from Drugs*, UICC Monograph Ser. 7, 48-52, Springer-Verlag, New York, 1967, 48.
28. Swenberg, J. A., Kostner, A., Wechsler, W., and Denlinger, R. H., Quantitative aspects of transplacental tumor induction with ethylnitrosourea in rats, *Cancer Res.*, 32, 2656, 1972.
29. Tomatis, L., Transplacental carcinogenesis, in *Modern Trends in Oncology*, Butterworths, London, 1973.
30. Vesselinovitch, S. D., Mihailovich, N., and Pietra, G., The prenatal exposure of mice to urethane and the consequent development of tumors in various tissues, *Cancer Res.*, 27, 2333, 1967.
31. Vesselinovitch, S. D., Comparative studies on perinatal carcinogenesis, in *Transplacental Carcinogenesis*, Scientific Publication No. 4, Tomatis, L. and Mohr, U., Eds., International Agency for Research on Cancer, Lyon, France, 1973, 14.
32. Vesselinovitch, S. D., personal communication.

SECTION 6
REPORT OF DISCUSSION GROUP NO. 5
INCLUSION OF POSITIVE CONTROL COMPOUNDS

John H. Weisburger

Public health statistics show that various forms of cancer constitute the second-largest cause of mortality in the United States, surpassed only by heart disease.[1] However, because of their often protracted terminal phases, neoplastic diseases actually constitute the most dreaded of human ailments. Various lines of evidence underwrite the concept that most types of cancer are due to environmental situations rather than a genetic, unavoidable factor.[18,21] Genetic factors only modulate the sensitivity of the response to a given environmental carcinogenic situation. Evidence that certain types of cancer are caused by specific chemicals comes from occupational observations where cancer followed exposure to some chemicals. Such cancers, while undesirable for the individuals concerned, amount, however, to only a small fraction of human cancers. That the major forms of human cancer, such as cancer of the colon, breast, and prostate, among others, are also due to mainly as yet unidentified chemical agents is adduced from studies of migrant populations going from a country or region of high incidence to one of low prevalence or vice versa.[4,5,8,9,21] Lung cancer, another major type of neoplasm, is due to excessive tobacco usage, discussed in detail by Dr. Hoffmann (see Section 7).

In order to make the environment safe from carcinogenic risks and, thus, prevent the occurrence and development of cancer, means are necessary to detect environmental agents with carcinogenic potential. These methods must not only be able to satisfactorily delineate a carcinogenic risk with pure chemicals, such as might be encountered in an occupational situation, but must also be able to assess such adverse effects with agents that might be responsible for the main human cancers noted above.

As is discussed in Sections 4 and 5, and as has been summarized in several reviews, currently used bioassay systems involve the administration of test chemicals or mixtures by suitable routes to animal systems, mostly rodents, namely mice, rats, and hamsters.[2,12,19]

In recent years, effort has centered on standard-izing such test systems and on relating them to each other as well as to newer in vivo and, indeed, in vitro assay procedures. The key to such standardization is the application of agents with known carcinogenic potential, the positive control compounds.

A positive control, thus, is a chemical with a known, reliable carcinogenic potential in a given test system. By this definition, when such a chemical is administered to a series of animals under exactly parallel conditions of procedural techniques, that is, species, strain, sex, and endocrine situation, starting age, and diet, it would be expected to produce a response that would be similar at diverse points in time. By this we mean that the average tumor incidence at a given target organ would be similar and that the latent period would be, by and large, identical. Any variation would need to be studied to delineate any deviation from the norm. Reproducibility under these conditions, with a known chemical carcinogen or, indeed, several different agents in a large-scale bioassay program, gives confidence that tests with unknown agents, which do or do not eventuate in a carcinogenic response, are also trustworthy.

As an example, in a small experiment where the active carcinogen N-hydroxy-N-2-fluorenylacet-amide was administered to hamsters at levels of 9 or 3 mg per kg per day, the animals' response was minimal. There was only an indication that higher doses or longer treatment might yield esophageal tumors. In view of this minimal response, it was decided that the null effects observed with several chemicals of unknown carcinogenicity being tested at the same time could not be relied upon with certainty. Thus, the failure of a positive control carcinogen to give a definite response created doubt about the validity of simultaneous tests of other chemicals where no carcinogenicity was seen.

Application of a positive control compound serves another useful purpose. Evaluation of the relative carcinogenic response with equal dose levels, when tested in different bioassay systems, permits conclusions to be drawn on the relative sensitivity of a given system to a particular class of chemicals. Because of the important differences in metabolic capability to produce active metabolites or detoxification products, discussed in Section 8, such generalizations and establishment of relationships are possible only within a restricted class of chemical agents.

Application of known carcinogens to the evaluation of newer in vitro systems, both in cell cultures, where the end point is transformed cells, or in mutagenicity assays, where the end point is mutant strains, needs to take into account the requirement for active metabolic systems leading to formation of proximate or ultimate carcinogen and also to detoxified products. To this end, the insertion of known carcinogens or their chemically prepared active intermediates offers a fruitful and, indeed, required means of standardizing the response of such systems.

A number of examples of positive control compounds in current use are listed in Table 1. In general, it is desirable that the positive control compound or compounds be chemically similar to the types of agent with unknown carcinogenic properties under test. It is desirable, although not mandatory, to use several dose levels of the positive control. The higher dose level would be certain to give the carcinogenic response rather quickly under the conditions of use. Lower dose levels might mimic a weaker response of unknown materials. Thus, the effect of an unknown material can be equated or related in a meaningful way to that of the known carcinogen at a given concentration, mode of administration, and other relevant procedural elements.

By current standards, interpretation of results of in vivo and in vitro bioassay programs will be facilitated if they include one or more positive control compounds. Since a properly selected agent will always give a response in a high yield relatively quickly, it may not be necessary to utilize large groups of animals, at least at the higher dose levels. For example, administration of adequate doses of diethylnitrosamine or of N-2-fluorenylacetamide reliably induces cancer in rodents. Groups of 15 to 25 are more than sufficient to check the reliability of the animal material. With unknown agents, group sizes two or three times as large will be necessary.

Bioassay programs involving oral administration of unknown test compounds, such as drugs, food additives, or industrial chemicals, are best accom-

panied by a positive control chemical yielding a high proportion of tumor-bearing animals with tumors at various sites, such as N-2-fluorenylacetamide and diethylnitrosamine among the powerful agents and 3-aminotriazole or safrole among the less potent carcinogens. For specific purposes, such as investigations of agents that might lead to stomach or colon cancer, N-methyl-N'-nitro-N-nitrosoguanidine has found favor. This latter chemical, being direct-acting and not requiring host-mediated metabolic activation, is also useful for in vitro systems, both in cell culture and mutagenicity tests.

The use in such tests of known carcinogens as positive controls does require the highest cleanliness and awareness of the potential hazards involved in handling of these agents. It is also true, however, that such principles need to be applied in any case, for the unknown chemicals or drugs tested may likewise be powerful carcinogens. Thus, the management of the test series, from the mixing and handling of the drugs or chemicals to the disposal of the residues, necessitates careful planning and execution. With respect to the disposal of residues, it can be said that the excreta from animals in most cases probably constitute minimal hazard, for the metabolites excreted are most likely of low carcinogenic risk. For disposal of organic combustible chemicals, bagging in plastic containers followed by complete incineration is recommended.

Another point deserving consideration is the fact that powerful carcinogens in a bioassay series would be discovered whether a positive control is used or not. Thus, for routine testing it is possible to conduct an adequate test without necessarily including a group treated with a known carcinogen. However, the example given above does suggest that negative results obtained in a test series, which at the same time document the sensitivity of the test system to a carcinogen, make a stronger case for drugs that are negative and thus give the appearance of safety.

During the deliberations of the group concerned with the assessment of the safety of drugs and discussing positive control carcinogens, it was concluded that the safety of drugs could be assessed with reasonable assurance, relative to the adequacy of results, without necessarily having a simultaneous test with a positive control carcinogen. It was felt, however, that a positive control might be desirable. It was further concluded that

TABLE 1

Typical Standard Carcinogens

Carcinogen	Species (strain)	Sex	Route	Dose	Main target organ and incidence	Latent period (weeks)	References
Diethylnitrosamine	Rat (Fischer)	M or F	Oral	40 ppm (in water)	Liver 100%	20	13, 20
Diethylnitrosamine	Rat (CR-SD)	M or F	Oral	51 ppm (in water)	Liver 100%	35	17
N-2-Fluorenylacetamide	Rat (CR-SD)	M	Oral	223 ppm (in diet)	Liver 90%	26–40	17
		M	Oral	80 ppm (in diet)	Liver 30%	60–90	Unpublished
		F	Oral	80 ppm (in diet)	Breast 50%	60–90	Unpublished
N-2-Fluorenylacetamide	Rat (Fischer)	F	Oral	2 mg (by gavage, 5 days per week)	Breast 20%	30–40	7
N-2-Fluorenylacetamide	Mouse	M or F	Oral	740 ppm	Liver	40	Unpublished
		M or F	Oral	240 ppm	Liver	90	Unpublished
Uracil mustard	Rat (Sprague-Dawley)	M	i.p.	11.5 mg/kg	Pancreas 4% Lymphoma 13% Peritoneum 22%	65 to death	6
		M	i.p.	23 mg/kg	Pancreas 8% Lymphoma 25% Peritoneum 33%	50 to death	6
		F	i.p.	11.5 mg/kg	Breast 55% Lung 10% Lymphoma 10% Peritoneum 10%	71	6
		F	i.p.	23 mg/kg	Breast 53% Lung 7% Lymphoma 14% Ovary 20% (0.5% controls) Peritoneum 40%	56	6

TABLE 1 (continued)

Carcinogen	Species (strain)	Sex	Route	Dose	Main target organ and incidence	Latent period (weeks)	References
Uracil mustard	Mouse	M or F	i.p.	0.008 g/kg	Lung 100%	24	16
		M or F	i.p.	0.020 g/kg	Lung 100%	24	16
		M or F	i.p.	0.040 g/kg	Lung 100%	24	16
Uracil mustard	Mouse	M	i.p.	9.3 mg/kg	Lung 64%	61 to death	6
		M	i.p.	19.3 mg/kg	Lung 50%	45 to death	6
		F	i.p.	9.3 mg/kg	Lung 60% Ovary 25% Lymphoma 50%	58	6
		F	i.p.	19.3 mg/kg	Lung 60% Ovary 33% Lymphoma 40%	69	6
Urethane	Mouse (A/He)	M or F	i.p.	10 mg	Lung 100%	24	16
		M or F	i.p.	20 mg	Lung 100%	24	16
N,N-Dimethyl-4-stilbenamine	Rat	M	Oral (in feed)	0.004%	Ear duct 63%	38	14a
3'-Methyl-4-dimethyl-aminoazobenzene	Rat	M	Oral (in feed)	0.05%	Liver 55%	37	14a
Nitrogen mustard	Mouse (A/J)	M or F	i.p.	0.21 mg/kg	Lung 40%	39	15
		M or F	i.p.	0.87 mg/kg	Lung 69%	39	15
		M or F	i.p.	3.4 mg/kg	Lung 95%	39	15
7,12-Dimethylbenz(a)-anthracene	Rat (SD)	F	Oral	15—20 mg (by tube)	Breast 92—100%	12—16	19
7,12-Dimethylbenz(a)-anthracene	Mouse	M or F	Skin	75 mg	Skin	10—25	3
3-Aminotriazole	Rat	M or F	Oral	300 ppm	Thyroid		14
		M	Oral	300 ppm	Liver 65%		14
		F	Oral	300 ppm	Liver 48% F		14

TABLE 1 (continued)

Carcinogen	Species (strain)	Sex	Route	Dose	Main target organ and incidence	Latent period (weeks)	References
3-Aminotriazole	Mouse (C57Bl/6XC3H/Anf)f$_1$	M or F	Oral	2,192 ppm	Thyroid Liver	78	10
Safrole	Rat (Osborne-Mendel)	M or F	Oral	5,000 ppm	Liver	104	11
	Mouse (C57Bl/6XC3H/Anf)f$_1$	M or F	Oral	1,112 ppm (in diet)	Liver	82	10

33

laboratories would be well advised to test the response of their bioassay systems at periodic intervals with properly selected positive controls.

In summary, present views on in vivo and in vitro bioassay procedures suggest that increased reliability and confidence accrue from the concurrent testing of an agent with a known carcinogenic response in the system. The agent needs to be carefully selected to relate meaningfully to other bioassay systems to permit semiquantitative interpretation of results with unknown agents and to assess the consistency of response of the systems selected. However, concern must be expressed that the use of such known, often powerful, carcinogens might involve possibly unnecessary exposure of laboratory personnel. Where carcinogens are involved in studies, stringent safety precautions must be taken to ensure that no contamination of staff, animals, or facilities arises. Specifically in relation to the bioassay of drugs, omission of a contemporary positive control series may be permissible. Nonetheless, under those conditions adequate assurance must be available, through periodic in-house tests, that positive responses are obtained with similar experimental protocols and animals by select standard carcinogens.

REFERENCES

1. Facts and Figures, American Cancer Society, New York, 1973.
2. Arcos, J. C., Argus, M. F., and Wolf, G., *Chemical Induction of Cancer,* Vol. 1, Academic Press, New York, 1968.
3. Bates, R. R., Sex hormones and skin tumorigenesis. I. Effect of the estrous cycle and castration on tumorigenesis by 7,12-dimethylbenz(*a*)anthracene, *J. Natl. Cancer Inst.,* 41, 559, 1968.
4. Berg, J. W., Haenszel, W., and Devesa, S. S., Epidemiology of gastrointestinal cancer, *Natl. Cancer Conf. Proc.,* 7, 459, 1973.
5. Doll, R., Environmental factors in the aetiology of cancer of the stomach, *Gastroenterologia,* 86, 320, 1956.
6. Griswold, D. P., Prejean, J. D., Casey, A. E., Weisburger, J. H., Weisburger, E. K., Wood, H. J., Jr., and Falk, H. L., Carcinogenicity studies of clinically used anticancer agents, *Proc. Am. Assoc. Cancer Res.,* 12, 65, 1971.
7. Hadidian, Z., Fredrickson, T. N., Weisburger, E. K., Weisburger, J. H., Glass, R. M., and Mantel, N., Tests for chemical carcinogens. Report on the activity of derivatives of aromatic amines, nitrosamines, quinolines, nitroalkanes, amides, epoxides, aziridines, and purine antimetabolites, *J. Natl. Cancer Inst.,* 41, 985, 1968.
8. Haenszel, W., Kurihara, M., Segi, M., and Lee, R. K. C., Stomach cancer among Japanese in Hawaii, *J. Natl. Cancer Inst.,* 49, 969, 1972.
9. Hirayama, T., Epidemiology of stomach cancer, *Gann Monogr.,* 11, 3, 1971.
10. Innes, J. R. M., Ulland, B. M., Valerio, M. G., Petrucelli, L., Fishbein, L., Hart, E. R., Pallotta, A. J., Bates, R. R., Falk, H. L., Gart, J. J., Klein, M., Mitchell, I., and Peters, J., Bioassay of pesticides and industrial chemicals for tumorigenicity in mice: A preliminary note, *J. Natl. Cancer Inst.,* 42, 1101, 1969.
11. Long, E. L., Nelson, A. A., Fitzhugh, O. G., and Hansen, W. H., Liver tumors produced in rats by feeding safrole, *Arch. Pathol.,* 75, 595, 1963.
12. Magee, P. N., Tests for carcinogenic potential, in *Methods in Toxicology,* Paget, G. E., Ed., F. A. Davis, Philadelphia, 1970, 158.
13. Magee, P. N. and Barnes, J. M., Carcinogenic nitroso compounds, *Adv. Cancer Res.,* 10, 163, 1967.
14. Napalkov, N., Influence of different functional activity of the thyroid gland on experimental carcinogenesis in the rat liver, in *Modern Problems of Oncology,* USSR Ministry of Health, Petrov Institute of Oncology, Leningrad, 1967, 78.
15. Shimkin, M. B., Weisburger, J. H., Weisburger, E. K., Gubareff, N., and Suntzeff, V., Bioassay of 29 alkylating chemicals by the pulmonary-tumor response in Strain A mice, *J. Natl. Cancer Inst.,* 36, 915, 1966.
16. Stoner, G. D., Shimkin, M. B., Kniazeff, A. J., Weisburger, J. H., Weisburger, E. K., and Gori, G. B., Test for carcinogenicity of food additives and chemotherapeutic agents by the pulmonary tumor response in Strain A mice, *Cancer Res.,* 33, 3069, 1973.
17. Ulland, B. M., Weisburger, J. H., Yamamoto, R. S., and Weisburger, E. K., Antioxidants and carcinogenesis: Butylated hydroxytoluene, but not diphenyl-*p*-phenylenediamine, inhibits cancer induction by N-2-fluorenylacetamide and by N-hydroxy-N-2-fluorenylacetamide in rats, *Food Cosmet. Toxicol.,* 11, 199, 1973.
18. Weisburger, J. H., Chemical carcinogenesis in the gastrointestinal tract, *Natl. Cancer Conf. Proc.,* 7, 465, 1973.
19. Weisburger, J. H. and Weisburger, E. K., Tests for chemical carcinogenesis, in *Methods in Cancer Research,* Vol. 1, Busch, H., Ed., Academic Press, New York, 1967, 307.
20. Williams, G. M. and Yamamoto, R. S., Absence of stainable iron from preneoplastic and neoplastic lesions in rat liver with 8-hydroxyquinoline-induced siderosis, *J. Natl. Cancer Inst.,* 49, 685, 1972.
21. Wynder, E. L. and Mabuchi, K., Etiological and preventive aspects of human cancer, *Preventive Med.,* 1, 300, 1972.

APPENDIX A TO REPORT OF DISCUSSION GROUP NO. 5
POSITIVE CONTROLS IN ENVIRONMENTAL RESPIRATORY CARCINOGENESIS

Dietrich Hoffmann and Ernest L. Wynder

During the past two decades, bioassays have been performed on the major respiratory pollutants, i.e., urban polluted air and tobacco smoke.[1,2] Several questions have arisen in these studies, which have necessitated the use of positive controls. These questions relate to comparisons of bioassay between different laboratories, to changes in carcinogenic potential of particulates with changes in precursors, and to the gradual modification in the source for these inhalants.

I. EXPERIMENTAL TOBACCO CARCINOGENESIS

During the last twenty years, significant modifications have occurred in the formation of commercial U.S. cigarettes. These include the use of different blends, changes in selection of tobacco varieties and tobacco strains, and the incorporation into the tobacco blend of midribs and stems, tobacco sheets, freeze-dried tobacco, and "flavoring agents." The effect of these changes on the carcinogenicity of the mainstream smoke, however, could only be observed by the use of positive controls (Figure 1).[3] These positive controls demonstrate that the susceptibility to carcinogens of the test organ, in this case mouse skin, has not

changed during the elapsed time and permits estimates concerning the carcinogenicity of cigarette smoke. Certainly, the observation of a reduction in tumorigenicity of tobacco smoke is most encouraging and indicates a positive trend towards the less harmful cigarette.

II. AIR POLLUTION CARCINOGENESIS

The particulate matter in polluted air originates primarily from incomplete combustions. These combustion products are relatively rich in polynuclear aromatic hydrocarbons (PAH) and include some known carcinogens. The question that arose is to what extent these carcinogenic hydrocarbons can explain the total carcinogenicity of the organic matter of urban pollutants. We have, therefore, tested the particulates together with benzo[a]pyrene (B[a]P) in four different concentrations as positive controls. By estimating the relative tumor potency for the test materials and positive controls, we were able to estimate the contribution of PAH, especially B[a]P, to the overall carcinogenicity of the air pollutants. By this method we were able to establish that between 40 and 60% of the carcinogenicity of the air pollution samples can be

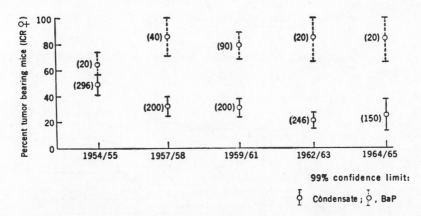

FIGURE 1. Decline of tumorigenicity, on mouse skin, of cigarette smoke condensates as tested during the period 1954-65 compared with the response to a 0.005% benzo[a]pyrene solution. Numbers in parentheses are numbers of mice per group. (Reprinted from Wynder, E. L. and Hoffmann, D., *Science*, 162, 862, 1968. With permission.)

explained by the presence of B[a]P alone (Figure 2), and it is estimated that all identified carcinogenic hydrocarbons are responsible for 60 to 80% of the total activity. This result suggests that the incomplete combustions are the major source of the carcinogenic potential of the polluted air in the three cities we studied, namely, Detroit, New York, and Los Angeles.

Frequently, the collection of air pollutants to perform a bioassay for complete carcinogenicity requires the filtering of very large volumes of air. In our own experience, even in such relatively polluted cities as Detroit and New York, the collection requires several weeks. Our earlier tests had demonstrated that polycyclic hydrocarbons can explain more than 50% of the total carcinogenicity of organic pollutants. Since the known carcinogenic hydrocarbons are all active as tumor initiators, and since the tumor initiator test requires relatively small amounts of PAH, we collected the particulates for only 24 hours and tested the organic matter for tumor-initiating activity with croton oil as tumor promoter (Figure 3). Again, the positive controls enabled us to evaluate the tumorigenic potential of relatively small samples of air pollutants. As for the complete carcinogenicity test, the presence of B[a]P can explain about 40 to 60% of the total activity.

III. RELATIVE CARCINOGENIC ACTIVITY OF PAH

In the past the carcinogenic potential of chemical agents, especially those of PAH, has been

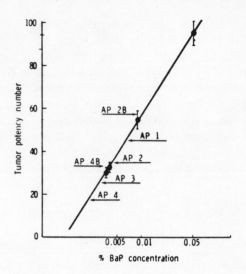

FIGURE 2. Method used for estimating the contribution of B[a]P to the tumorigenicity of organic air pollutants. (Reprinted from Wynder, E. L. and Hoffmann, D., *Tobacco and Tobacco Smoke,* Academic Press, New York, 1968, 730. With permission.)

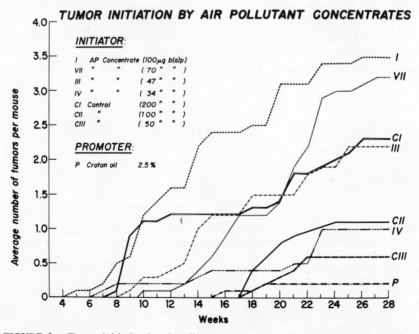

FIGURE 3. Tumor initiation by air-pollutant concentrates. (Reprinted from Wynder, E. L. and Hoffmann, D., *Tobacco and Tobacco Smoke,* Academic Press, New York, 1968, 730. With permission.)

TABLE 1

Chrysene and Methylchrysenes: Tumor-initiating Activity[a]

Promoter application (weeks)	No. of mice with tumors	Total tumors	Survivors	Promoter application (weeks)	No. of mice with tumors	Total tumors	Survivors
Chrysene				**4-Methylchrysene**			
1	0	0	20	1	0	0	20
10	0	0	19	10	0	0	20
12	1	1	18	12	2	2	20
14	3	6	18	14	2	2	20
16	6	9	18	16	3	3	20
18	8	15	18	18	7	9	20
20	11	19	18	20	7	9	20
1-Methylchrysene				**5-Methylchrysene**			
1	0	0	20	1	0	0	20
10	0	0	20	10	3	3	19
12	0	0	20	12	6	9	19
14	2	2	19	14	12	31	19
16	2	2	19	16	13	49	19
18	5	5	19	18	17	92	18
20	6	6	19	20	17	96	18
2-Methylchrysene				**6-Methylchrysene**			
1	0	0	20	1	0	0	20
10	0	0	19	10	0	0	19
12	0	0	19	12	1	1	19
14	2	2	19	14	1	1	19
16	6	9	19	16	5	8	19
18	8	13	19	18	7	11	19
20	8	13	19	20	7	11	19
3-Methylchrysene				**Benzo[a]pyrene**			
1	0	0	20	1	0	0	20
10	0	0	20	10	0	0	20
12	1	1	20	12	1	1	20
14	3	5	20	14	4	5	20
16	6	11	20	16	6	9	20
18	11	21	20	18	6	10	20
20	14	26	20	20	6	10	20

[a]Female, Swiss albino mice (Ha/1CR/Mil) were used. The tumor initiator dose for chrysene and the methylchrysenes was ten applications of 0.1 mg in 1 ml of acetone, and that for benzo[a]pyrene was ten applications of 0.0005 mg in 1 ml of acetone. The tumor promoter dose was 2.5 μg of TPA, given three times weekly. The acetone controls were negative.

Reprinted from Hoffmann, D., Bondinell, W. E., and Wynder, E. L., *Science*, 183, 215, 1974. With permission.

TABLE 2

Carcinogenic Activity of the 3-, 5-, and 6-Methylchrysenes[a]

Application (weeks)	3-Methylchrysene			5-Methylchrysene						6-Methylchrysene				B[a]P		
	Total no. of mice	Tumors		Total no. of mice	All tumors		Carcinoma			Total no. of mice	All tumors			Total no. of mice	Tumors	
		No. of mice	Total No.		No. of mice	Total No.	No. of mice	Total No.			No. of mice	Total No.			No. of mice	Total No.
1	20	1	1	20						20				20		
11	20	1	1	20	3	3				20				20		
15	20	1	1	20	7	13				19				20		
20	20	1	1	19	18	64	5	5		19	2	2		20	1	1
25	19	1	1	16	20	85	9	11		19	2	2		20	1	1
30	18	1	1	12	20	99	12[b]	37		19	2	2		20	3	4

[a]The methylchrysenes were given three times a week in doses of 0.1 mg in 0.1 ml of acetone; benzo[a]pyrene (B[a]P) was given in a dose of 0.005 mg in 0.2 ml of acetone. Under the conditions described, chrysene, 1-methylchrysene, 2-methylchrysene, and 4-methylchrysene showed no activity.

[b]The eight mice that were killed had carcinomas, which were histologically confirmed. Two mice had multiple metastases in the lung and spleen. In the eight mice examined histologically (20 to 30 weeks of treatment), we did not find any lung adenomas or any primary tumors other than skin papillomas and carcinomas.

Reprinted from Hoffmann, D., Bondinell, W. E., and Wynder, E. L., *Science*, 183, 216, 1974. With permission.

indexed with one to four plus signs.[4] Whereas these plus signs can serve as a guideline, they are only of limited value for estimating the contribution of individual carcinogens to the overall activity of an environmental factor. We have, therefore, always correlated the carcinogenicity and tumor-initiating activity of active agents to positive controls.

We would like to explain this technique on a sample of our current studies.[5] Tobacco smoke contains relatively high concentrations of alkylated chrysenes. We tested, therefore, the six possible methylchrysenes and chrysene itself together with B[a]P. In the case of tumor-initiating activity we applied 1.0 mg of chrysene or of one of the methylchrysenes and 0.005 mg of B[a]P as initiator, and tetradecanoyl phorbol acetate (TPA) as promoter. The assay was completed after 20 weeks of promoter application (Table 1) and suggested that in this setting only 1.0 mg of 3-methylchrysene and 1.0 mg of 5-methylchrysene have significantly higher tumor-initiating activity than 0.05 mg of B[a]P. At present we are testing these three hydrocarbons in three different doses in order to estimate their relative tumor-initiating activity.

For the complete carcinogenicity assay we tested the chrysenes in 0.1% concentration and B[a]P as positive control in 0.005% concentration. After only 20 to 30 weeks we have found that 5-methylchrysene is a powerful carcinogen, whereas the other chrysenes are weak or inactive carcinogens with activities not exceeding that of the low B[a]P concentration (Table 2). This experiment demonstrates that with the positive control we save time and material, since we have only to test 5-methylchrysene in different concentrations to estimate its carcinogenic potential.

SUMMARY

Positive controls are essential in performing a bioassay for carcinogenicity of environmental agents, since they enable us to check constantly and over many years the reproducibility of our bioassay system. Positive controls also enable us to estimate the relative carcinogenic potency of an environmental agent or synthetic chemical. Bioassay data from tobacco carcinogenesis, air pollution carcinogenesis, and from the bioassay of some carcinogenic polycyclic hydrocarbons were presented for demonstrating the importance of positive controls.

REFERENCES

1. **Hoffmann, D. and Wynder, E. L.,** Chemical analysis and carcinogenic bioassays of organic particulate pollutants, in *Air Pollution,* Stern, A. C., Ed., Academic Press, New York, 1968, 187.
2. **Wynder, E. L. and Hoffmann, D.,** *Tobacco and Tobacco Smoke,* Academic Press, New York, 1968, 730.
3. **Wynder, E. L. and Hoffmann, D.,** Experimental tobacco carcinogenesis, *Science,* 162, 862, 1968.
4. **Schoental, R.,** Carcinogenesis by polycyclic aromatic hydrocarbons and certain other carcinogens, in *Polycyclic Hydrocarbons,* Vol. 1, Clar, E., Ed., Academic Press, New York, 1964, 133.
5. **Hoffmann, D., Bondinell, W. E., and Wynder, E. L.,** Carcinogenicity of methylchrysenes, *Science,* 183, 215, 1974.

SECTION 8
INTERPRETATION OF TEST RESULTS
IN TERMS OF CARCINOGENIC POTENTIAL TO THE TEST ANIMAL:
THE REGULATORY POINT OF VIEW

William D'Aguanno

The evaluation of safety in laboratory animals should include a definition of the toxicity of the potential drug and the circumstances under which toxicity is manifested. In the initial stages of this evaluation, there is usually an interdigitation of studies in experimental animals and man. As clinical studies progress, additional animal data are developed to support broader clinical trials and, ultimately, to support the general availability of the drug to the medical community. It is at this point that one can assess the predictive value of the animal and determine the degree of correlation between animals and man for most toxicological effects.

Carcinogenesis differs from many other kinds of toxicity in that it is an irreversible response that may involve a long latent period between chemical insult and pathological manifestation. This is one of the factors that makes it difficult to monitor carcinogenicity in humans. For drugs inducing this effect, animal studies are particularly important in determining a benefit—risk ratio.

Although chemical carcinogenesis was discovered in humans two centuries ago (scrotal cancer in chimney sweeps, by Sir Percival Pott), the first experimental induction of cancer with a pure chemical compound was not achieved until 1930. Since then, studies on the causation and prevention of cancer have shown about 1,000 chemicals capable of producing cancers in experimental animals, and 20 to 30 substances are known to produce cancers in man. With the exception of the arsenicals, all those chemicals reported to induce human cancer have also proved oncogenic in one or more species of lower animals. Given the present state of surveillance of the use of drugs by man and the difficulties inherent in both human monitoring and retrospective epidemiological studies, tests in laboratory animals still provide the major evidence bearing on the possible carcinogenicity of a drug.

In drug-safety evaluation, a tumorigen is defined as a substance that, when administered by an appropriate route, causes an increased incidence of tumors in experimental animals as compared to a control series of untreated animals. The response to a tumorigenic substance may consist of (1) an increased incidence of tumors of a type seen commonly in the control animals, (2) the development of a type of tumor not seen in the control animals, or (3) a combination of the occurrence of a different type of tumor and an increased incidence of one or several types of tumors seen in the controls. In some experiments the only manifestation of an effect consists of (4) an earlier occurrence of tumors in the treated animals than in the controls, the incidence being the same in both. In yet another variation the only effect seen may consist of (5) an increase in the number of tumors per animal, the number of tumor-bearing animals being the same. Any one of these effects may suggest the presence of a carcinogenic hazard. The word "tumor" is, in this context, defined as a neoplastic lesion, usually seen grossly as a new nodular tissue formation. A distinction is generally made between benign tumors and malignant tumors. Strictly speaking, these terms relate to the ultimate fate of the organism carrying the tumors. Malignant lesions present clear-cut evidence for the presence of the disease, whereas the rate of growth and the biochemical and morphological properties of benign tumors often approximate those of normal tissues. The word "carcinogen" is reserved only for drugs causing tumors that are malignant or that are strongly suspected of progressing from the benign to the malignant state.

The question of whether benign tumors always progress to malignant ones is controversial. An excess of benign tumors over their incidence in vehicle or untreated controls is interpreted as an abnormality. When there is reliable evidence that a compound induces benign tumors under certain experimental conditions, a great deal of suspicion becomes attached to the compound. Where justified by the practical or theoretical importance of the compound, additional tests in different strains or species, in younger animals, or by different routes of administration might be indicated.

One difficulty in determining the relevance of animal studies to humans is that the susceptibility of different species to a given tumorigen or carcinogen shows considerable variation. A carcinogen that is active in one species may vary in effect in different species in terms of target organ or may be totally inactive in other species, e.g., β-naphthylamine. The susceptibility of a species may also depend on the genetic strain of the animal, sex, dietary conditions, route of administration, and even the solvent or "carrier vehicle."

The evaluation of laboratory data should include a consideration of the pathogenesis of the observed effects, whether the tumor arose either as a direct insult to the genetic apparatus of the cell or as a result of other tissue changes often involving an increased turnover of cells.

Radiomimetic drugs and irradiation are agents probably characteristic of the first type of effect. In the other category, the tumors produced are probably secondary to other lesions. Griseofulvin, for example, interferes with porphyrin metabolism in the liver of the mouse, leading to an accumulation of material and changes in the parenchyma with subsequent tumor formation.[1,5] The metabolic change does not occur in man at therapeutic doses, and it is therefore unlikely that tumors will occur in man by a mechanism similar to that in mice.[7]

There is evidence in many cases of apparent chemically induced tumors that concretions may be a factor in carcinogenesis. Fitzhugh and Nelson[3] stated that "in all but one instance of tumor in weanling rats, stones were also present in the bladder, pointing very strongly to the factor of chronic irritation in the production of tumors." Weil et al.[8] reported that bladder tumors never developed without the preceding or concurrent presence of a foreign body. In man, however, little or no relationship has been found between bladder stone and tumor formation.

As a general rule, the time required for tumor induction in any species depends on its total life span. Even the most potent carcinogens require periods measured in months in mice and rats, species with an average life span of 18 months and three years, respectively. The minimal period required to induce effects in animals with potent agents ranges from 1/8 to 1/4 of the life span.

In any safety evaluation program both the design of the experimental protocol and the method of analysis or interpretation of resulting data must be considered; the experimental design should not be established apart from the plan for analysis of data. In tests for potent carcinogens relatively few animals may be needed. The situation becomes more complex and the interpretation proves more difficult when agents are tested for weak carcinogenic effect. Under these conditions only a small fraction of the animals at risk may be affected, and the latent period may be so long as to be in the range where control animals also show tumors.

Use of laboratory animals for carcinogenic assay requires reliance on a method with relatively low sensitivity, in comparison with the degree of sensitivity we would desire. The factor that limits sensitivity is usually the number of test animals used. For example, an observed outcome of no tumors in a group of 100 test animals and 100 negative controls provides assurance at the 99% probability level that the tumor risk is under 4.5%. It would require tumor-free results in 450 animals to establish with equal probability that the degree of risk is below 1%. Experiments of this dimension would overwhelm both the investigator and the laboratory in most cases. This is particularly so because of the need for continuous observation and careful examination of organs and tissues by highly qualified personnel.

The determination of minimum effective doses and the whole concept of "threshold dose" have been the subject of considerable discussion in recent years in the context of dose—response relationships in chemical carcinogenesis. The question is whether or not there exists a "safe" subthreshold dose, or rate of intake, of carcinogenic chemicals. Based on the persistence of effect and the additive effect of repeated doses for a sufficiently long time, some investigators conclude that no "safe" dose for carcinogenic substances may be set. The problem of existence of biological threshold has been discussed by Dinman.[2] Using the suggestion that 10^4 drug molecules per cell is the limiting concentration for biological activity, Friedman[4] calculated 8.6×10^{15} molecules per kilogram of cells as the minimum number to evoke a biological effect.

A different analysis, based on statistical considerations, of the concept of threshold dose was made by Mantel and Bryan.[6] They concluded that the carcinogenic hazard never disappears, but gradually becomes smaller with diminishing dose. They suggest as a practical approach not to attempt a determination of threshold level, but rather to determine a "socially acceptable" or arbitrarily safe level. The authors further qualify their recommendation by the recognition that such arbitrary "safe" levels can become unsafe when certain noncarcinogenic compounds are present that enhance the potency of the carcinogenic agent. This is analogous to the determination of a benefit–risk ratio while recognizing that the ratio is not a constant. Rather, new information acquired from clinical investigation and usage, additional animal studies, or development of other therapeutic agents could result in a shift in the ratio.

While the general operating policy and priorities for carcinogenicity testing used by the Food and Drug Administration have evolved primarily over the past decade, they are not dissimilar from those recommended in the reports of a scientific committee of the World Health Organization.[9] The operating policy is based on a number of factors, such as the nature of the disease to be treated, the life expectancy of the patient, the age of the patient population, the pharmacological activity of the agent, species differences in drug disposition and metabolism and, of course, availability of other therapeutic agents, all of which are the factors used in calculating the benefit–risk ratio.

A candidate substance for long-term testing is one that is placed in the "suspect" category either by reason of its chemical similarity to substances known to induce tumors or on the basis of information on its biological activity obtained in the course of general safety testing. Additionally, drugs used by large segments of the population and those likely to be administered for prolonged periods are considered to be candidates for carcinogenicity screening.

Some drugs should be tested during the early stages in the development of a new drug, while others may be studied during the later stages.

1. Drugs to be tested before they are given to man: Among the compounds considered here would be those "suspected" carcinogens that suggest an unacceptable benefit–risk ratio. It is generally agreed that such compounds would include those chemically related to a known carcinogen. Chemicals that exhibit adverse effects on rapidly growing tissues in short-term experiments or that affect mitosis are usually included in this category also.

2. Drugs to be tested during clinical trial: Drugs to be administered for prolonged periods as well as those for which broad population exposure is anticipated should be tested during the clinical trial stage if they have not been previously tested.

3. Drugs to be tested after release for marketing: For selected new drugs it may be determined that carcinogenicity testing is needed, but this should not delay marketing. Drugs in this category would include those of medical importance where a benefit–risk determination favors rapid availability of the drug for patient care. In such cases restricted labeling may be needed until the situation is clarified by completion of testing.

4. Drugs on the market that should be tested: Many drugs currently marketed have not been subjected to long-term tests nor evaluated for carcinogenic hazard. A preliminary study has been initiated to determine the extent of the problem and the assignment of priorities for these drugs.

In establishing these priorities, consideration has been given to a number of limitations imposed by the activity of many of the new drugs, the time-consuming animal bioassay with low sensitivity, the limitation of qualified personnel and resources, and the ratio of compounds undergoing clinical investigation to compounds that finally become marketed drugs.

Utilizing the limited resources to greatest advantage is certainly an important consideration. More meaningful studies in animals can be performed from the standpoint of dosage selection, species selection, and even the need for a study if the therapeutic value, dosage, and metabolism of the drug are known in man. Detection of tumorigenic responses in animals should be considered an opportunity for further research. If a determination is made that a chemical has elicited a carcinogenic response, elucidation of its mechanism and metabolism should be attempted.

The welfare of patients and prevention of exposure to unnecessary risk is our common objective. The interpretation of data requires a sensitivity to benefit–risk considerations. In regulating the development and marketing of drugs, it is important that FDA policies and guidelines reflect the current state of scientific knowledge, and that they undergo continuing review to reflect scientific developments in a rapidly changing field.

REFERENCES

1. **Barich, L. L., Schwarz, J., Barich, D. J., and Horowitz, M. G.,** Toxic liver damage in mice after prolonged intake of elevated doses of griseofulvin, *Antibiot. Chemother.,* 11, 566, 1961.
2. **Dinman, B. D.,** "Non-Concept" of "No-Threshold": Chemicals in the environment, *Science,* 175, 495, 1972.
3. **Fitzhugh, O. G. and Nelson, A. A.,** Comparison of the chronic toxicity of triethylene glycol with that of diethylene glycol, *J. Ind. Hyg. Toxicol.,* 28, 40, 1946.
4. **Friedman, L.,** Problems of evaluating the health significance of the chemicals present in foods, *Pharmacology and the Future of Man,* Proceedings of the Fifth International Congress on Pharmacology, San Francisco, 1972, Vol. 2, Karger, Basel, 1973, 30.
5. **Hurst, E. W. and Paget, G. E.,** Protoporphyrin, cirrhosis and hepatomata in the livers of mice given griseofulvin, *Br. J. Dermatol.,* 75, 105, 1963.
6. **Mantel, N. and Bryan, W. R.,** "Safety" testing of carcinogenic agents, *J. Natl. Cancer Inst.,* 27, 455, 1961.
7. **Rimington, C., Morgan, P. N., Nicholls, K., Everall, J. D., and Davies, R. R.,** Griseofulvin administration and porphyrin metabolism, *Lancet,* 2, 318, 1963.
8. **Weil, C. S., Carpenter, C. P., and Smythe, H. F.,** Urinary bladder response to diethylene glycol, *Arch. Environ. Health,* 11, 569, 1965.
9. Principles for the Testing and Evaluation of Drugs for Carcinogenicity, *Technical Report Series,* No. 426, World Health Organization, Geneva, 1969.

SECTION 9
INTERPRETATION OF TEST RESULTS
IN TERMS OF SIGNIFICANCE TO MAN

Philippe Shubik

In the 1969 report of a World Health Organization scientific group on the Principles for the Testing and Evaluation of Drugs for Carcinogenicity,[1] certain basic definitions were proposed that, I believe, can serve as useful guidelines for discussion of my topic "Interpretation of Results in Terms of Significance to Man." At the outset of the report, a most important distinction was made between four different situations, namely:

1. Drugs to be tested before they are administered to man: These are compounds considered to be so potentially hazardous as a result of their chemical structure or biological characteristics that it is considered unwise to administer them to man even in clinical trials.

2. Drugs that should be tested during clinical trials: There may be some special requirements (drugs to be given for prolonged periods or to pregnant women) that provide for some of the characteristics required for carcinogenic action in the absence of other special features.

3. Drugs that should be tested after marketing: This is a blanket category of drugs that should be tested routinely, without special reasons, unless carcinogenicity can be ruled out. (Is this ever possible?)

4. Drugs on the market that should be tested: In this instance there are some cases in which epidemiological data have come to light that suggest that carcinogenicity may exist, or some of the other criteria may apply.

Each of these situations clearly provides different sets of facts that may be used to determine the basis for extrapolation to man.

There is a series of questions that are asked repeatedly in the context of interpretation of significance to man. Most often these questions have been asked in terms of problems concerning evaluation of the safety of food additives. This is a much more restricted situation, and many of the features that occur in the instance of drugs do not apply or are just not available for contemplation. Most food additives have not been evaluated in man, and indeed, apart from their usefulness in terms of their particular function, they probably cannot be so evaluated.

In the majority of instances the metabolism of given drugs has been well evaluated in man, and certain of the major hurdles in extrapolation have been overcome. Meaningful epidemiological studies are often possible with drugs. This situation is hard to envisage in the instance of most food additives, not absolutely impossible, of course, but, nevertheless, most unlikely.

To start with, I should like to confine my assessment to that situation in which the primary problem concerns the extrapolation of "conventional" animal data to man. The most important question is whether or not a particular test is "appropriate" for the particular use conditions of the drug in question. There is a series of obvious questions to be asked that must be answered not in absolutes but rather in terms of leeway permitted.

If the study is to be performed in animals, obviously the first question is whether or not the animal used is the appropriate one. Here the different categories play a major role. Obviously, it might be possible in the instance of a drug that is already past some of its clinical trials to use knowledge of its metabolic patterns in man to select an appropriate test animal. If it is not possible to do this in depth, it may at least be possible to avoid entirely unsuitable circumstances. In most instances it seems impossible to find the appropriate animal, and it is still usual to use more than one species in an effort to extend the parameters of the test. Clearly, a knowledge of the metabolism of the drug is an important, if not vital, consideration in the extrapolation of any test. If the compound is not metabolized similarly in the experimental animal and in man, I believe that the investigator should hesitate to extrapolate his results. On the other hand, if there is no information of the metabolic pathway of the compound in man available, we are, of course, forced to ignore this parameter and assume that it might well be the same. In the instance in which the compound is negative in one species and positive in another or others, there would seem to be good *prima facie* evidence that the metabolism of the compound to a "proximate" carcinogen is probably an important factor. In this instance it would seem to me that the only proper course to adopt is to attempt to elucidate the matter scientifically. As much information as possible should be obtained on the metabolic pathways before extrapolating for practical purposes in the instance of a drug that has clearly apparent beneficial effects.

At this point a purist might point out that we do not know the chemical mechanism of action of any carcinogen, that any of the metabolic pathways under discussion may, indeed, be found irrelevant to carcinogenesis. Since most carcinogenic chemicals yield a range of metabolic products, there seems little doubt that some of these are merely the products of usual pathways of detoxification and may have no significance to carcinogenesis. It may be that the final "proximate" carcinogen will only represent a minute fraction of the compound administered.

The second question that I shall address concerns the route of administration of the compound. Obviously, an appropriate test of a drug should involve the same route of administration in the experimental animal as that used in man. In many discussions on carcinogenesis testing for various purposes the matter of route of administration is variously discussed. It has been suggested that two routes of administration should be used to obviate possible metabolic differences between the test animal and man and to extend the parameters of the test.[1] Although there is some merit to this approach, much caution must be exercised in extrapolating from certain routes of administration to others.

It is my personal belief that the cardinal rule must be that the test mimic conditions of use as much as possible. In general, a drug only administered orally should be tested by the same route of administration. Of course, many medications are given by different routes, and in such cases all of the different routes should be investigated in the test if it seems logical. We are periodically faced with a situation where some investigator may have tested one drug or another by a route of administration that is different from that used in practice. Common sense should prevail in extrapolating such results. In other areas of toxicology much

difficulty has been engendered in the past by tests using the subcutaneous route of administration for compounds used orally (e.g., food dyes).[2] No one can say that the subcutaneous route of carcinogenesis is meaningless as an indicator; however, there is no doubt that many such tests merely reflect the physical nature of the injection rather than the chemical effects and cannot be extrapolated.

In recent years there has been much emphasis on the transplacental route of administration.[3] Carcinogenesis tests are begun in the F_0 generation and studied in the F_1. Clearly, such findings have considerable relevance to the use of drugs in pregnant women. Can these findings be extrapolated to humans in general? The transplacental system appears to be more sensitive to the effects of certain carcinogens than the adult. Perhaps this is only in regard to certain tumors. As with the administration of carcinogens to the newborn,[4] it is indeed difficult to make meaningful quantitative comparisons. Not only does one have to take into account different numbers of tumors and their latent periods; in addition, the differences in tumor types are of major importance. It is difficult to make a pronouncement in this instance and to say, merely because a test reveals carcinogenicity only in the transplacental system and none in the adult, that the findings are only relevant to the human transplacental situation. The interpretation of the studies in this instance may call into play either enhanced susceptibility of the system in general or a specific effect applying only to the transplacental system. Only additional study can solve this problem. At this point, however, one must point to the desirability of performing transplacental studies in all instances where such exposure may occur. In summary, therefore, extrapolation of animal data to man in the instance of drugs should, in general, call for use of similar routes of administration. However, on some occasions, where carcinogenicity may have been demonstrated by some other method, careful analysis of the system is needed and, on occasion, additional studies.

The problem of dosage will be dealt with in my third point. The question of "safety margin" in the testing of food additives has been variously interpreted. In most instances, the Food and Drug Administration rule of thumb employing 100-fold exaggeration for the dose with a no-effect level has, it would seem to me, served us well. In the instance of carcinogenicity testing, the usually accepted procedure has been to use the maximal tolerated dose as the highest dose level in the test animals. The definition of this level with precision is not easy, nor is it easy to detect the meaning in the literature. In the minds of some investigators, maximal tolerated dosage implies that no change occurs at this level even on chronic feeding. Others believe that minimal toxic effects, such as weight loss, should be detected at top levels. The report of the World Health Organization group suggests that the high levels should be within the toxic range.[1] Although I was a member of the World Health Organization group and subscribed to this view at that time, I have changed my mind and would prefer to see tests performed at dosages below the toxic range. I believe that the primary consideration here should be the nature of the toxic side effects induced. I do not know with certainty of any side effects that can be related to the induction of malignancies. I do, however, believe that there is a series of situations in which such interrelationships may be suspected and that there is a series of situations in which some induced "side effect" would make the test quite unrealistic. The induction of bladder calculi would certainly be a factor in determining the induction of neoplasms of the bladder. This might occur only at levels high enough to bring about changes in mineral balance, which would not be seen at all at doses within the range recommended for practical purposes. Certain hormonal carcinogens must be tested at dose ranges that provide proper physiological backgrounds. There is the problem of the "pill," which can be evaluated properly only in relationship to the menstrual cycle and which at high dosages in rodents will induce irrelevant side effects.

In the instance of food additives, we are often faced with a situation in which we are testing an agent that is to be ingested by millions of people, often at a relatively low level. In the instance of most drugs (although by no means all), we are faced with a situation in which often relatively few people will be treated, usually with relatively high dosage levels, calculated to bring about therapeutic effects. It is, therefore, the case that drugs may give rise to certain detectable biological effects that are part and parcel of their desired effects, and that the test procedure can be made close to reality.

As with any toxicity testing procedure, we must, of necessity, introduce safety margins to compensate for the fact that our test population of animals will be well below the numbers dealt with in the treated human population. The primary method for achieving this is by increasing the dosage of the compound. It must be borne in mind that the test may be inappropriate at the higher levels as a result of side effects.

In this general context it must be mentioned that the precise mode of administration is most important and that administration in drinking water rather than mixed with food, in various solvents, by gavage, etc., may introduce other factors of considerable importance in extrapolating to man.

My fourth point concerns the matter of numbers. It is quite essential that some concept of the level of statistical significance aimed at be known prior to the start of the experiment, and that test groups and control groups be of adequate size to permit such determinations. In recent years one can point to several studies in carcinogenesis that have been used for regulatory purposes where "suggestive trends not statistically significant" have been pointed out. I do not believe that any scientist has any business making such a statement. There are experiments that have suggested further experiments to many of us. We do the experiments and comment later. I do not know what the appropriate level of significance should be in general and believe that it must vary considerably, depending on the nature of the drug to be tested. In the instance of the pill, for example, I believe that we should demand studies providing us with as high a level of significance as practically possible. With life-saving antibiotics given for relatively short periods, I believe that lower levels are acceptable. Most studies aim at a P (probability) value of 0.05. This seems practical within the present structure of society, and the alteration of these standards clearly demands an analysis of many factors, including certain sociological considerations.

Whatever else can be said, I do believe that we have reasonably objective methods for assessing "statistical significance." Tests not meeting these requirements should not be extrapolated to man. Once statistical significance has been established, it should be considered in the context of the particular practical example under study and form part of the final evaluation. It cannot be an absolute measure alone.

For my fifth point I should like to consider some of the special features of the response in the carcinogenicity test. The word "carcinogen" can be defined in a series of different ways. I have come to believe in recent years that the term should be dropped, since it now encompasses such a large range of different agents acting in some instances in microgram quantities (aflatoxins), in some cases in milligram quantities, and in still others in gram quantities (aromatic amines), and including some agents, such as the hormonal carcinogens, that cause neoplasms only after inducing many preliminary effects. The response in the experimental animal may be a striking one in which some tumors not seen or hardly seen in the controls occur in massive numbers in the treated animals, or the response may merely be one in which the test compound causes an increased number and lowered latent period for the tumors seen commonly in untreated control animals. The fact that our control animals do not, in practice, have well-controlled environments (animal feeds, for example, used in most studies are not semisynthetic but rather commercial mixtures of unknown composition) and have many neoplasms of totally unknown origin makes one realize that our pronouncements are based on less than satisfactory scientific data.

To any logical observer there would seem to be a difference between these responses. However, in our present state of ignorance, we cannot make a distinction. I, for one, worry much more about a compound that induces a range of new tumors than one that enhances the lung adenoma incidence in mice. One has a tendency to feel that perhaps the hepatoma of the mouse is not an indicator of such potential hazard to man as, for example, the induction of bladder tumors in dogs. I do not know whether this is so. I believe that many more facts are needed before the decision can be based upon scientific grounds. For the time being, I think that one can only use both indices as indicative of potential hazard and use common sense and all the facts available to make a final determination.

I should like, at this point, to introduce three examples from our own studies to illustrate some of these points. These are isoniazid (INH), metronidazole, and griseofulvin.

In the instance of INH, the first reports indicated that both lung adenoma and lymphoma incidences were increased.[5] Subsequent investi-

gations have demonstrated that INH administration inhibits the occurrence of mammary tumors in C3H mice.[6] The lung adenoma effect has been confirmed many times. However, the lymphoma-induction effect has not been substantiated.[7] INH is not carcinogenic in the hamster.[8] It has been reported to induce hepatomas in an isolated instance in the rat,[9] but this has not been substantiated.[10-12] The carcinogenic action of this compound in animals is, therefore, limited indeed. Studies on the metabolic pathways of the compound have been undertaken in an effort to elucidate these differences but are not complete. Initial studies suggested that hydrazine was the active metabolite. This has not been confirmed, although, as a result of this suggestion, many hydrazine derivatives are now known to be highly carcinogenic. (I say highly because they induce many tumors not reported in control animals, of the colon, for example.) According to various sources, 50 to 90% of INH is metabolized to 1-acetyl-1-isonicotinoylhydrazine in man. This compound has recently been shown by my colleague, Dr. Toth,[13] to be carcinogenic in mice, inducing lung adenomas.

Wisely, I believe, these results had no effect on the use of INH in tuberculosis in any respect, including the prophylactic use of the compound. I hope, however, that proper steps are being taken to follow these human cases prospectively, so that some data may eventually be obtained that will enable us to extrapolate with confidence. For the moment, the additional metabolic studies comparing the mouse and hamster data with man may provide the basis for reasonable judgment.

In our studies with metronidazole the situation is reasonably similar. We have found that this drug increases the incidence of lymphomas and lung adenomas in mice.[14] We have negative results in the hamster. The compound might be suspected to be a potential carcinogen from its chemical structure. Metabolism studies are needed, and human prospective studies should be made. The drug is used for different purposes. In one instance it is used as a trichomonicide, and in another for the control of amebiasis. In the latter instance, the use of the drug as a life-saving medication should, in my view, not be regulated. In the case of its use as a trichomonicide, it might be prudent to consider substituting other methods for controlling a benign condition.

The last example is a study that is not

complete, involving griseofulvin. Griseofulvin has been known for some years to give rise to hepatomas in mice.[15] It has additional effects, e.g., inducing porphyria, that might well be much more important than this carcinogenic action. It is the only good antifungal agent, and any suggestion that it might be banned cannot be considered. Our approach has been to study this compound in additional species. The mouse study has been repeated and confirms prior findings;[16] the rat and the hamster seem negative thus far. Again, the best approach is, of course, to set up prospective studies in man and to undertake any metabolism studies possible — a difficult, if not impossible, problem in this instance.

Last of all, I should like to raise one question that I do not propose to answer in toto. "What measures of competence are there in experimental performance of such studies? How can one conclude that the study was a good, reliable one?"

There are certain characteristics of the facility in which the study was performed that are known to all of us and should be closely noted. Personally, I am most disturbed by the approach taken to pathological examination of tissues. I do not believe that it is possible to perform proper studies in carcinogenesis without the full participation of a trained pathologist. The specimens must be taken by the pathologist himself or by a technician directly under his supervision. It is not possible to perform such studies properly when the pathological diagnosis must be done in another institution.

I believe that it is high time to develop standard criteria for the licensing of toxicological laboratories. No evaluation in terms of extrapolation to man can be meaningful unless full confidence exists in the standards of the investigation. I regret having to say this, but realistically most toxicologists agree that such confidence is necessary. Extrapolation from conventional animals to man

has to be carefully considered. I have pointed here only to some of the most obvious limitations.

However, I cannot conclude without mentioning other types of study. Rapid-test methods have been well reviewed. Tissue-culture methods are discussed widely; we are investigating their use ourselves, but have not settled on any particular method. For the moment they can be no more than screening procedures to be used prior to thorough animal investigations. The use of studies for mutation has been mentioned frequently. Again, the fact that a compound is mutagenic certainly suggests that it should be thoroughly tested for carcinogenicity.

The occurrence of carcinogenicity from use of a drug can surely mean that certain drugs would be more of a risk than a benefit. In other cases the situation may be reversed. Each case must be studied in depth before a decision can be made, and often the result will be the planning of additional studies. The most pressing need at the present time is for better human surveillance of those agents shown to be carcinogenic in animals.

The history of iatrogenic cancer makes us look upon this area with great caution. There is no doubt in my mind that there is more potential hazard present in this field than any other. This is because the amounts of chemical administered for therapeutic purposes tend to be high and, by comparison with food additives, are another order of magnitude. Our animal test methods can only provide us with a warning. They cannot predict effects in another species with absolute certainty in most cases. Our judgment thus must take many facts into account. Better methods are needed, but for the moment I think that we are not testing adequately even within present methodology and not giving enough consideration to some of the potential hazards that have been drawn to our attention.

REFERENCES

1. WHO Scientific Group on Principles for the testing and evaluation of drugs for carcinogenicity, *W.H.O. Tech. Rep. Ser.*, No. 426, 1969.
2. Joint FAO/WHO Expert Committee on Food Additives, Specifications for the identity and purity of food additives and their toxicological evaluation: Some emulsifiers and stabilizers and certain other substances, *W.H.O. Tech. Rep. Ser.*, No. 373, 1967.
3. Food and Drug Administration Advisory Committee and Protocols for Safety Evaluation, Panel on carcinogenesis report on cancer testing in the safety evaluation of food additives and pesticides, *Toxicol. Appl. Pharmacol.*, 20, 419, 1971.
4. Toth, B., A critical review of experiments in chemical carcinogenesis using newborn animals, *Cancer Res.*, 28, 727, 1968.
5. Juhász, J., Balo, J., and Kendrey, G., Az isonikotinsavhydrazid (INH) daganatkelto hatasanak kiserletes vizsgalata, *A Tuberkulozis*, 3–4, 49, 1957.
6. Toth, B. and Shubik, P., Mammary tumor inhibition and lung adenoma induction by isonicotinic acid hydrazide, *Science*, 152, 1376, 1966.
7. Toth, B. and Shubik, P., Carcinogenesis in Swiss mice by isonicotinic acid hydrazide, *Cancer Res.*, 26 (Part 1), 1473, 1966.
8. Toth, B. and Shubik, P., Lack of carcinogenic effects of isonicotinic acid hydrazide in the Syrian golden hamsters, *Tumori*, 55, 127, 1969.
9. Severi, L. and Biancifiori, C., Hepatic carcinogenesis in CBA/Cb/Se mice and Cb/Se rats by isonicotinic acid hydrazide and hydrazine sulfate, *J. Natl. Cancer Inst.*, 41, 331, 1968.
10. Toth, B. and Toth, T., Investigations on the tumor producing effect of isonicotinic acid hydrazide in AWS/Sn mice and MRC rats, *Tumori*, 56, 315, 1970.
11. Pansa, E., Picco, A., and Gravi, M., Sul problema del supposto effetto carcinogenetico dell'idrazide dell'acido isonicotinico (IAI). Ricerche sperimentali sul ratto, *Minerva Med.*, 53, 3162, 1962.
12. Peacock, A. and Peacock, P. R., The results of prolonged administration of isoniazid to mice, rats, and hamsters, *Br. J. Cancer*, 20, 307, 1966.
13. Toth, B. and Shimizu, H., Lung carcinogenesis with 1-acetyl-2-isonicotinoylhydrazine, the major metabolite of isoniazid, *Eur. J. Cancer*, 9, 285, 1973.
14. Rustia, M. and Shubik, P., Induction of lung tumors and malignant lymphomas in mice by metronidazole, *J. Natl. Cancer Inst.*, 48, 721, 1972.
15. Unpublished data.
16. Unpublished data.

SECTION 10
CARCINOGENIC EFFECTS OF DRUGS IN MAN

Joseph F. Fraumeni

The identification of chemical agents that cause cancer has come largely from studies in laboratory animals and surveys of industrial workers. In contrast, only limited information is available on drugs as carcinogens in man. The evidence was recently reviewed by Fraumeni and Miller[1] and is summarized in Table 1.

Radioisotopes exert carcinogenic effects by release of ionizing radiation at deposition sites in the body. For example, radioactive phosphorus (^{32}P) increases the risk of leukemia in patients with polycythemia vera.[2] Radium and mesothorium, bone-seeking isotopes once used for various illnesses, produced a high rate of osteogenic sarcoma and carcinoma in mucous membranes near bone, such as the paranasal sinuses.[3] The same effect resulted from occupational exposures among radium-dial painters and radium chemists. Thorotrast, deposited in the reticuloendothelial system after use in radiographic studies, induced hepatic hemangioendotheliomas in many cases.[4]

Immunosuppressive agents (antilymphocyte serum, antimetabolites, corticosteroids) have been suspected as contributing factors to the high cancer risk reported in renal transplant recipients, perhaps by inhibiting immunologic surveillance that ordinarily limits the progression of initiated or transformed cells. In a recent follow-up study of 6,297 recipients of kidney transplants, the risk

TABLE 1

Cancers Related to Drug Exposures in Man

Radioisotopes

Phosphorus (^{32}P)	Acute leukemia
Radium, mesothorium	Osteosarcoma and sinus carcinoma
Thorotrast	Hemangioendothelioma of liver

Immunosuppressive drugs (for renal transplantation)

Antilymphocyte serum	Reticulum cell sarcoma
Antimetabolites	(?) Other cancers (skin, liver, soft-tissue sarcoma)
Corticosteroids	

Cytotoxic drugs

Chloronaphazine	Bladder cancer
Melphalan	
Cyclophosphamide	Acute myelomonocytic leukemia

Hormones

Synthetic estrogens	
Prenatal	Vaginal and cervical adenocarcinoma (clear-cell type)
Postnatal	Endometrial carcinoma (adenosquamous type)
Androgenic-anabolic steroids (for aplastic anemia)	(?) Hepatocellular carcinoma

Others

Arsenic	Skin cancer
Phenacetin-containing drugs	Renal-pelvis carcinoma
Diphenylhydantoin	(?) Lymphoma
Coal-tar ointments	Skin cancer
Chloramphenicol	(?) Leukemia

of developing lymphoma was about 35 times normal expectation and derived almost entirely from a risk of reticulum-cell sarcoma that was 350 times higher than expected.[5] Skin and lip cancers occurred up to 4 times more often than expected, whereas the risk of other cancers showed a 2½-fold excess in men only, due largely to soft-tissue sarcoma and hepatobiliary carcinoma. Since persons with heritable immune-deficiency syndromes are susceptible to lymphoma and possibly other cancers,[6] it is likely that immunosuppressive drugs play a role in post-transplant carcinogenesis. However, there is no evidence that cancers develop excessively in other conditions treated with these drugs, so that the predisposition may result from interaction between immunosuppression and immunostimulation by antigens from the grafted kidney.

Cytotoxic agents used in cancer chemotherapy are often carcinogenic in laboratory animals, and some may induce cancer in man.[7] Chlornaphazine was withdrawn in 1964, when high doses for polycythemia vera and Hodgkin's disease were found to cause bladder tumors.[8] This drug is a derivative of β-naphthylamine, which was known to be a bladder carcinogen in industrial workers. In addition, certain alkylating agents seem to elevate the risk of acute leukemia, especially the myelocytic and monomyelocytic types. Most striking has been an increase in leukemia among patients with multiple myeloma treated with melphalan or cyclophosphamide,[9] although one cannot yet exclude the possibility that improved survival has permitted the development of a hematopoietic neoplasm related to the origin or natural history of myeloma. Another effect of cytotoxic drugs was suggested by a recent follow-up study of Hodgkin's disease, which showed that intensive chemotherapy enhanced the risk of second cancers originating at heavily irradiated sites.[10]

Synthetic estrogens, particularly stilbestrol, have triggered much recent concern about the carcinogenic effects of drugs. First evidence for a human transplacental carcinogen came in 1971, when a link was reported between stilbestrol and a cluster of vaginal adenocarcinoma among eight women in Boston between 14 and 22 years of age.[11] Retrospective study showed that the mothers of seven of the eight girls were treated with stilbestrol during pregnancy to prevent miscarriage. These findings were confirmed by study of a similar case cluster reported to the cancer registry of New York State.[12] At present, prenatal exposure to synthetic estrogens has been linked to clear-cell carcinomas of the vagina and cervix in dozens of patients ranging from 7 to 25 years in age.[13] Since the risk of cancer is greatest after puberty, it is possible that endogenous estrogens are involved in promoting tumor development. The observations in man are consistent with experimental studies showing the heightened susceptibility of embryos and newborn animals to carcinogens.[14,15]

Synthetic estrogens given after birth may also induce cancer. In a recent study of 24 patients receiving stilbestrol over a period of at least five years for gonadal dysgenesis, endometrial carcinoma developed in two, and possibly in three, cases.[16] Together with three cases in the literature, the tumors were diagnosed in patients between 28 and 35 years of age, and most were of an unusual mixed or adenosquamous type. In addition, cancers of the breast have been reported to be excessive in men receiving stilbestrol for prostatic cancer; however, the tumors now appear not to be primary in the breast, but metastases from the prostate.[17]

Exogenous androgens have been implicated in a recent series of four patients with hepatocellular carcinoma following long-term treatment of aplastic anemia with androgenic-anabolic steroids, primarily oxymetholone or methyltestosterone derivatives.[18] Additional cases have been reported[19] and underscore the need for further evaluation of these compounds.

Inorganic arsenicals have not been shown to be carcinogenic in experimental animals. However, when taken internally, the agents are generally considered to cause skin cancer in man.[20,21] The skin cancers following use of arsenicals are characteristically multiple, involve unexposed parts of the body and unusual locations (e.g., palms of the hands), and are associated with arsenical pigmentation and hyperkeratosis. Instances of lung cancer and liver hemangioendothelioma have been attributed to medicinal arsenic, but these occurrences may be chance.[21]

Large doses of analgesic drugs containing phenacetin are a causal factor in chronic pyelonephritis and papillary necrosis. Reports from Sweden and, recently, from Australia indicate that patients with "analgesic nephropathy" are at high risk of developing transitional-cell tumors of the renal pelvis.[22,23] It is surprising that this complication has not been reported in the United States or other countries; further studies are obviously needed.

Diphenylhydantoin (Dilantin) is an anticonvulsant drug that occasionally induces lymphoid reactions that regress on cessation of therapy. Transformation of this state to malignant lymphoma has been reported in several patients.[24] The nature of this association remains to be defined, but recent evidence in man and laboratory animals suggests that the drug may predispose to lymphoma by its capacity to concurrently depress and stimulate immune responses.[25,26]

Coal-tar and creosote preparations (containing polycyclic hydrocarbons) have been reported to cause skin cancer in laboratory animals, in exposed workers, and in patients using the preparations.[27]

Chloramphenicol and other marrow-depressing drugs have been implicated by case reports in the development of leukemia.[28,29] A causal relationship would be consistent with the potential of leukemogenic agents (radiation, benzene, alkylating agents) to produce aplastic anemia.[29,30] The production of chromosomal defects by chloramphenicol[31] supports the possibility of a leukemia hazard, since such defects are seen in various conditions at high risk of leukemia.[30]

Future approaches to the study of drug-induced cancer, as discussed recently,[1] are outlined in Table 2. One outcome of this conference would be to improve the lines of communication between experimentalists and epidemiologists. In general, the epidemiologist influences laboratory investigations of drug-induced cancer by contributing leads from human observations, and by testing hypotheses that evolve from the laboratory. Thus, opportunities for research by epidemiologists and experimentalists are greatly enhanced by developments in either field. Consideration should be given to the formation of channels for transmitting research developments from one field to another.

TABLE 2

Future Investigations of Drug-induced Cancers in Man

1. Laboratory studies
2. Surveillance of trends
3. Alert clinicians
4. Retrospective studies
5. Prospective studies
6. Special-disease registries
7. Record-linkage systems
8. Study of early-life exposures
9. Interdisciplinary communication

REFERENCES

1. Fraumeni, J. F., Jr. and Miller, R. W., Drug-induced cancer, *J. Natl. Cancer Inst.*, 48, 1267, 1972.
2. Modan, B. and Lilienfeld, A. M., Leukaemogenic effect of ionising-irradiation treatment in polycythaemia, *Lancet*, 2, 439, 1964.
3. Hasterlik, R. J. and Finkel, A. J., Diseases of bones and joints associated with intoxication by radioactive substances, principally radium, *Med. Clin. North Am.*, 49, 285, 1965.
4. da Silva Horta, J., Cayolla da Motta, L., Abbatt, J. D., and Roriz, M. L., Malignancy and other late effects following administration of thorotrast, *Lancet*, 2, 201, 1965.
5. Hoover, R. and Fraumeni, J. F., Jr., Risk of cancer in renal transplant recipients, *Lancet*, 2, 55, 1973.
6. Gatti, R. A. and Good, R. A., Occurrence of malignancy in immunodeficiency diseases, *Cancer*, 28, 89, 1971.
7. Ryser, H. J.-P., Chemical carcinogenesis, *N. Engl. J. Med.*, 285, 721, 1971.
8. Thiede, T., Chievitz, E., and Christensen, B. C., Chlornaphazine as a bladder carcinogen, *Acta Med. Scand.*, 175, 721, 1964.
9. Kyle, R. A., Pierre, R. V., and Bayrd, E. D., Multiple myeloma and acute myelomonocytic leukemia. Report of four cases possibly related to melphalan, *N. Engl. J. Med.*, 283, 1121, 1970.
10. Arseneau, J. C., Sponzo, R. W., Levin, D. L., Schnipper, L. E., Bonner, H., Young, R. C., Canellos, G. P., Johnson, R. E., and DeVita, V. T., Nonlymphomatous malignant tumors complicating Hodgkin's disease, *N. Engl. J. Med.*, 287, 1119, 1972.

11. Herbst, A. L., Ulfelder, H., and Poskanzer, D. C., Adenocarcinoma of the vagina: Association of maternal stilbestrol therapy with tumor appearance in young women, *N. Engl. J. Med.*, 284, 878, 1971.
12. Greenwald, P., Barlow, J. J., Nasca, P. C., and Burnett, W. S., Vaginal cancer after maternal treatment with synthetic estrogens, *N. Engl. J. Med.*, 285, 390, 1971.
13. Herbst, A. L., Kurman, R. J., Scully, R. E., and Poskanzer, D. C., Clear-cell adenocarcinoma of the genital tract in young females. Registry report, *N. Engl. J. Med.*, 287, 1259, 1972.
14. Napalkov, N. P., Some general considerations on the problem of transplacental carcinogenesis, in *Scientific Publication No. 4*, Tomatis, L. and Mohr, U., Eds., International Agency for Research on Cancer, Lyon, France, 1973, 1.
15. Vesselinovitch, S. D., Comparative studies on perinatal carcinogenesis, in *Scientific Publication No. 4*, Tomatis, L. and Mohr, U., Eds., International Agency for Research on Cancer, Lyon, France, 1973, 14.
16. Cutler, B. S., Forbes, A. P., Ingersoll, F. M., and Scully, R. E., Endometrial carcinoma after stilbestrol therapy in gonadal dysgenesis, *N. Engl. J. Med.*, 287, 628, 1972.
17. Benson, W. R., Carcinoma of the prostate with metastases to breasts and testis. Critical review of the literature and report of a case, *Cancer*, 10, 1235, 1957.
18. Johnson, F. L., Lerner, K. G., Siegel, M., Feagler, J. R., Majerus, P. W., Hartmann, J. R., and Thomas, E. D., Association of androgenic-anabolic steroid therapy with development of hepatocellular carcinoma, *Lancet*, 2, 1273, 1972.
19. Henderson, J. T., Richmond, J., and Sumerling, M. D., Androgenic-anabolic steroid therapy and hepatocellular carcinoma, *Lancet*, 1, 934, 1973.
20. Lee, A. M. and Fraumeni, J. F., Jr., Arsenic and respiratory cancer in man: An occupational study, *J. Natl. Cancer Inst.*, 42, 1045, 1969.
21. IARC *Monograph on the Evaluation of the Carcinogenic Risk of Chemicals to Man: Some inorganic and organometallic compounds*, Vol. 2, International Agency for Research on Cancer, Lyon, France, 1973, 48.
22. Bengtsson, U., Angervall, L., Ekman, H., and Lehmann, L., Transitional cell tumors of the renal pelvis in analgesic abusers, *Scand. J. Urol. Nephrol.*, 2, 145, 1968.
23. Taylor, J. S., Carcinoma of the urinary tract and analgesic abuse, *Med. J. Aust.*, 1, 407, 1972.
24. Anthony, J. J., Malignant lymphoma associated with hydantoin drugs, *Arch. Neurol.*, 22, 450, 1970.
25. Kruger, G., Harris, D., and Sussman, E., Effect of Dilantin in mice. II. Lymphoreticular tissue atypia and neoplasia after chronic exposure, *Z. Krebsforsch.*, 78, 290, 1972.
26. Grob, P. J. and Herold, G. E., Immunological abnormalities and hydantoins, *Br. Med. J.*, 2, 561, 1972.
27. Rook, A. J., Gresham, G. A., and Davis, R. A., Squamous epithelioma possibly induced by the therapeutic application of tar, *Br. J. Cancer*, 10, 17, 1956.
28. Fraumeni, J. F., Jr., Bone marrow depression induced by chloramphenicol or phenylbutazone. Leukemia and other sequelae, *J. Am. Med. Assoc.*, 201, 828, 1967.
29. Fraumeni, J. F., Jr., Clinical epidemiology of leukemia, *Semin. Hematol.*, 6, 250, 1969.
30. Fraumeni, J. F., Jr. and Miller, R. W., Epidemiology of human leukemia: Recent observations, *J. Natl. Cancer Inst.*, 38, 593, 1967.
31. Cohen, H. J. and Huang, A. T., A marker chromosome abnormality. Occurrence in chloramphenicol-associated acute leukemia, *Arch. Intern. Med.*, 132, 440, 1973.

SECTION 11
REPORT OF DISCUSSION GROUP NO. 7
SPONTANEOUS TUMORS AND RELATED PATHOLOGIC CHANGES

R. K. Bickerton

I. INTRODUCTION

In the testing of any potential drug for carcinogenicity, the appearance of spontaneous tumors in the test species assumes major significance in the interpretation or evaluation of the data. Many reports describing the incidence of spontaneous tumors occurring in various species have been written. It is not the intent of this document to reiterate or even extend these tables, but rather to discuss briefly certain aspects of the occurrence of spontaneous tumors as they relate to the evaluation of the carcinogenic potential of chemicals.

II. GENERAL CONSIDERATIONS

Although the major portion of this document will be devoted to the occurrence of spontaneous tumors and related pathologic changes in various species, certain factors are important in all species and thus can be considered independently.

The determination whether a drug is a carcinogen depends upon one or more of the following criteria:

1. Increased tumor incidence;
2. A decrease in the latency of tumor appearance;
3. Appearance of tumors in organs where spontaneous tumors did not occur.

Assessment of each of these requires comparison of results obtained in treated animals to those obtained in concurrent controls. As such, detailed knowledge of the occurrence of spontaneous tumors is essential. This is particularly true when tests for weak carcinogens extend over the lifetime of the species. It would be ideal if the appearance of a tumor as a function of time could be plotted for each organ. For easily detected tumors (i.e., skin, mammary gland) such practice is quite feasible; however, for tumors of internal organs it is quite difficult. It is nonetheless important, and in experiments terminated at earlier than life span, recording only of overall tumor incidence may not allow accurate assessment of which, if any, of the three criteria were affected. Simple comparison at one point in time of tumor incidence in animals with spontaneous tumors and those treated with drugs may lead to erroneous conclusions in assessing the effect of the chemical.

Many factors can influence the reported incidence of spontaneous tumors. For example, nutritional, endocrine, immunologic, and environmental status all can alter the spontaneous incidence. Dietary restriction, for example, has been shown to reduce the incidence of spontaneously occurring mammary tumors in Sprague-Dawley rats. Conversely, increasing the lipid component of a diet has been shown to increase th incidence of spontaneous mammary tumors in the rat. Similarly, in mice, Tannenbaum[A-1] has shown that, following exposure to a carcinogen under good dietary conditions, a reduced tumor incidence occurs if the animals are subsequently given a diet lacking in essential factors.

Natural or artificially induced alteration in levels of various hormones can affect the incidence of spontaneous tumors. Specifically, the administration of large amounts of estrogen leads to mammary or pituitary tumors in animals. The high incidence of spontaneous mammary tumors in female rats may be dependent upon very definite ratios of estrogen to progesterone; this ratio is distinctly different in rats than it is in man. Further, the reduction in spontaneous mammary-tumor incidence in the female Sprague-Dawley rat as a result of ovariectomy or adrenalectomy is well known. Environmental factors, such as lighting and nutrition, may alter endocrine patterns. The influence of such altered endocrine patterns on the development of spontaneous tumors in animals must be considered.

The demonstration that induced tumors are antigenic, together with the demonstration that young animals with immature immune systems are more sensitive to carcinogenic chemicals, testifies to the importance of immunologic factors in the development of spontaneous as well as of induced tumors. Indeed, the differences in spontaneous-tumor incidences in various strains of animals may be due to immunologic differences. As such, the immunologic status of the animal might be an important consideration in assessing the spontaneous-tumor incidence.

As mentioned above, various environmental factors can influence the incidence of spontaneous tumors in various species of animals, some of these presumably through alteration in endocrine patterns. Other environmental factors are equally important. Such items as control of temperature and humidity are obvious. Equally obvious is the need for general cleanliness in rooms containing animals under investigation. The existence of infectious or noninfectious concomitant diseases, which may or may not shorten the life span of the animal, can also affect the incidence of spontaneous tumors. The number of animals per cage can affect the incidence of spontaneous tumors, particularly in small animals. Also, environmental contaminants, such as DDT, aflatoxin and other known carcinogens (such as those used as positive controls), and asbestos particles from air-conditioning filters may elicit tumors in control groups.

For the reasons outlined above, in the testing for carcinogenicity of new drugs, it is important to assess the spontaneous-tumor incidence in adequate numbers of control animals housed and handled identically and concurrently with the treated group. Animals should be randomly assigned to treatment and control groups.* Data on spontaneous-tumor incidence are of value, particularly in the selection of the species when low or high spontaneous incidence of certain tumors is desired. It is also important in selecting strains susceptible to chemical carcinogens.

III. SPECIFIC SPECIES

Because of ease and economy in handling adequate numbers of animals, the mouse and the rat have been the most frequently used animals in the assessment of a chemical for carcinogenic potential. In view of this, emphasis in this document will be given to discussion of spontaneous tumors and related pathologic changes in the mouse and the rat. This is not meant to imply that other species are not useful or, indeed, that they should not be used, but rather reflects current practice. There are instances where selection of a species other than rodent would be more appropriate, and in this instance it is hoped that the discussion on spontaneous tumors and related pathologic changes in other species will be useful.

A. Rat

Many strains of rats have been used in tests for carcinogenicity. For the purposes of this document, the discussion will emphasize animals derived from the Sprague-Dawley rat and the Fischer-344 rat, since these seem to be the two most widely used.

It seems to be well documented that most strains of rat have a relatively high incidence of spontaneous tumors, particularly the older animals. (For a detailed survey, the reader is referred to Volume I of *Methods in Cancer Research*.)

A wide variety of spontaneous tumors are seen in most strains of rat. Table 1 gives a listing of tumors and the percentage incidence observed in a lifetime (90% mortality) study in a group of Charles River Sprague-Dawley rats and a group of Fischer-344 rats.† Data in a similar format are reported in the publications of Hadidian et al. (1966) and Ribelin and McCoy (1965) for Fischer rats, and of Shubik et al. (1962), Davis et al. (1956), and Durbin et al. (1966) for Sprague-Dawley rats.

The tumor occurring with the highest frequency in both sexes of both strains was pituitary adenoma. It has been reported that pituitary adenoma is often a finding at autopsy in female rats showing mammary tumors. While there is a high incidence of pituitary adenoma in both the Sprague-Dawley and the Fischer rat, there is not a one-to-one correlation. Mammary tumors are seen in rats in which no pituitary adenomas could be detected at autopsy or in histopathologic examination. There does not seem to be a direct cause-and-effect relationship. Further, male rats show a rather high incidence of pituitary adenoma (though only 50% of the incidence seen in females), and yet few mammary tumors are seen.

*Sampling procedures have been demonstrated to affect the reported incidence of spontaneous neoplastic lesions (Thompson, S. and Hunt, R., *Ann. N.Y. Acad. Sci.*, 108, 832, 1963; Thompson, S., *Lab. Invest.*, 28, 398, 1973).

†Housed under excellent living conditions (Norwich Pharmacal Co., unpublished).

TABLE 1

Characteristic Spontaneous Tumors in the Sprague-Dawley and Fischer Rat

Tumor	Sprague-Dawley M	Sprague-Dawley F	Fischer M	Fischer F
Percent incidence (from 50 animals of each sex)				
Skin				
Verruca vulgaris			2	
Squamous-cell carcinoma	2		2	
Apocrine adenoma			2	2
Sebaceous adenoma			4	2
Malignant sebaceous adenoma			2	
Dermis				
Fibrosarcoma		2		
Dermal fibroma	8	6	4	
Leiomyosarcoma				2
Leiomyoma		2	2	
Mammary Gland				
Intraductal adenoma		2		
Adenoma	4	22	6	8
Adenofibroma	2	44		34
Adenocarcinoma		2		2
Adenoma with carcinomatous tendency		2		
Neural				
Neurofibroma	2			
Malignant neurofibroma			2	
Astrocytoma	2			
Urogenital				
Ovarian arrhenoblastoma		2		
Urocystic papilloma	4		2	
Interstitial-cell tumor – testes	2		60	
Uterine leiomyoma				6
Renal pelvic papilloma		2		
Prostatic carcinoma			2	
Renal-cell carcinoma			2	
Endocrine				
Pituitary adenoma	24	72	22	50
Pheochromocytoma	2		6	
Sympathicoblastoma	14		6	
Adrenal cortical adenoma		8		
Thyroid light cell	6	6	8	12
Pancreatic islet cell	2	4		2
Adrenal ganglioneuroblastoma				2
Thyroid Hurtle cell	2			
Thyroid adenoma		2		

TABLE 1 (continued)

Tumor	Percent incidence (from 50 animals of each sex)			
	Sprague-Dawley		Fischer	
	M	F	M	F
Gastrointestinal				
Gastric leiomyosarcoma	2			
Abdominal mesothelioma			4	
Cardio-respiratory				
Angiosarcoma with metastasis		2		
Bronchial adenoma				4
Lymphoreticular				
Leukemia	2		24	6
Lymphosarcoma	4	4	6	2
Reticulum-cell sarcoma			2	
Malignant histiocytosis			2	
Histiocytic sarcoma with metastasis	2			
Histiocytic sarcoma without metastasis		2		
Cartilage, Bone, Muscle				
Chondroma	2			
Rhabdomyosarcoma	2			
Periosteal fibroma	2			

Courtesy Norwich Pharmacal Co.

However, it would not be surprising, in view of the known pituitary influence on the mammary gland, to find a relationship to tumor development in some animals. This would seem to offer a fruitful area for further research.

In the female of both strains the mammary gland shows a high percentage of spontaneous tumors. But there is a marked difference in mean time of appearance (16 months in Sprague-Dawley, 22 months in Fischer rats). The paper by Durbin et al. (1966) gives valuable data on variability of occurrence of tumor types. This variability must be considered in assessing the carcinogenic potential of drugs.

In addition to the pituitary adenoma mentioned above, a variety of other endocrine tumors are observed in both strains in significant numbers. These include thyroid, pancreatic, and adrenal tumors. In the male Fischer rat, there is a high frequency of spontaneous interstitial-cell testicular tumors; this tumor is not frequently observed in Sprague-Dawley rats. Other tumors occur in small numbers and with much variability. As such, one might expect drug-treated animals to show some sporadic tumors not seen in controls when the tumors were in fact not drug-induced. The finding of a small percentage of tumors in treated animals (in organs where their occurrence has been demonstrated) versus no percentage in control animals should not implicate the drug as a carcinogen. However, a low frequency of occurrence of tumors in organs where spontaneous tumors are not seen should implicate the drug for further study (e.g., one tumor of the glandular stomach).

The use of the Long-Evans rat as well as that of other strains is increasing. There is a need to have data from detailed lifetime studies on spontaneous-tumor incidence in these strains and others as well to insure proper interpretation of studies in carcinogenicity.

The occurrence in large numbers and the

variability in latency of spontaneous mammary tumors and endocrine tumors in the Sprague-Dawley and Fischer rats and of testicular tumors in the Fischer rat, as well as a wide variety of spontaneous tumors in other organs, make interpretation of tests for carcinogenicity of drugs extremely difficult. It would seem ideal to search for a rodent species that has high sensitivity to chemical carcinogens but low spontaneous incidence of tumors. In the interim, however, it seems the only solution is to study more than one strain of rat. Comparison of tumor incidences among strains should ease the complex task of the evaluation.

B. Mouse

The inbred mouse has been widely used in research. Dunn, in a chapter on "Spontaneous Lesions of Mice," has listed various qualities that make it a valuable laboratory animal.[B-1] They are

1. Mice are relatively inexpensive to purchase and maintain.

2. The mouse has a short life span.

3. Voluminous literature has been accumulated on the normal and pathologic anatomy, physiology, endocrinology, and many biochemical reactions of the mouse.

4. The mouse is the smallest of the commonly used laboratory animals.

5. Many inbred strains have been developed, and most of them are readily available.

The choice of strain to be used is most important. For assistance in making the choice, investigators are referred to "Standardized Nomenclature for Inbred Strains of Mice: Fifth Listing" (*Cancer Res.*, 32, 1609, 1972). Valuable information on the spontaneous occurrence of tumors in mice is to be found in Tables 2, 3, and 4.

References on the morphology of spontaneous tumors in laboratory mice were selected from a list[B-2],[B-5] compiled by the Registry of Experimental Cancers.

The references compiled by the Registry are available in easily accessible journals or

TABLE 2

Some Suggested Inbred Strains for Studies of Neoplasms

Neoplasm	Strains	Incidence of neoplasm
Mammary-gland tumors	C3H	Almost 100% in ♀♀
	A	High in breeding ♀♀, low in virgin ♀♀
	DBA	High in breeding ♀♀
	RHI	High in breeding ♀♀
	BALB/c	Incidence low, but high following introduction of mammary-tumor agent
	CC57BR CC57W	Do not develop spontaneous mammary tumors; 55% after introduction of mammary-tumor agent
Pulmonary tumors	A	90% in mice living to 18 months
	SWR	80% in mice living to 18 months
	BALB/c	26% in ♀♀, 29% in ♂♂
	BL	26% in mice of all ages
Hepatomas	C3H	85% in males 14 months old
	C3Hf	72% in males 14 months old
	C3He	78% in males 14 months old 91% in breeding ♂♂; 59% in virgin ♀♀; 30% in breeding ♀♀; and 38% in force-bred ♀♀
Leukemia and other reticular-cell neoplasms	C58	High leukemia
	AKR	High leukemia
	C57L	Hodgkins-like lesion, reticular-cell neoplasm Type B, approximately 25% at 18 months

TABLE 2 (continued)

Neoplasm	Strains	Incidence of neoplasm
Papilloma and carcinoma of skin	HR	Papillomas occurred in all mice, both haired and hairless, painted with methylcholanthrene, and the carcinomatous transformation occurred in most of the animals
	I	Most susceptible of 5 strains tested with methylcholanthrene
Subcutaneous sarcomas	C3H	Occurred spontaneously in 57 of 1774 C3H and C3Hf ♀♀
		Most susceptible of 8 strains tested with carcinogenic hydrocarbons
	CBA	High occurrence after subcutaneous injection of methylcholanthrene
Stomach lesion	I	Occurs in practically all mice of this strain
	BRS BRSUNT }	Occurs following injection with methylcholanthrene and spontaneously
Adrenal cortical tumors	CE	High occurrence following castration
	NH	High occurrence of spontaneous adenoma
		High occurrence of carcinoma following castration
Teratomas, testicular	129	1%, congenital
Interstitial-cell tumors of testis	A	Readily induced with estrogens
	BALB/c	High incidence following treatment with stilbestrol (males tolerate stilbestrol better than do those of other strains)
Pituitary adenoma	C57BL	Occurred in almost all mice treated with estrogens
Hemangioendotheliomas	HR	19 to 33% in untreated mice
		54 to 76% in mice injected with 4-o-tolylazo-o-toluidine
	BALB/c	High occurrence, particularly in interscapular fat pad and lung in mice treated with o-aminoazotoluene
Ovarian tumors	C3He	47% in virgin ♀♀; 37% in breeding ♀♀; 29% in force-bred ♀♀
Myoepitheliomas	A BALB/c	Occur in region of salivary gland and clitoral gland
Harderian gland tumors	C3H	Occur in C3H and hybrids resulting from outcrossing C3H

From Heston, W. E., Genetics of neoplasia, in *Methodology in Mammalian Genetics,* Burdette, W. J., Ed., Holden-Day, San Francisco, 1963, 249. With permission.

TABLE 3

Characteristic Tumors of Inbred Strains, Sex, and Age Incidence

Tumor type	Strain	Incidence (%)	Type of mouse	Average age (months)
Mammary-gland tumor	C3H	99	Breeding ♀ ♀	7.2
		100	Virgin ♀ ♀	8.8
	DBA/2	77	Breeding ♀ ♀	15
		Lower	Virgin ♀ ♀	
	A	84	Breeding ♀ ♀	
		5	Virgin ♀ ♀	
	DD	84	Breeding ♀ ♀	7.7
		75	Virgin ♀ ♀	10.2
Lymphocytic leukemia	AKR	92		8.0
	C58	90		10.0
Primary lung tumor	A	90		After 18
	SWR	80		After 18
Hepatoma	C3HeB	91	Breeding ♂ ♂	21.4
		58	Virgin ♀ ♀	24.1
		30	Breeding ♀ ♀	21.0
Reticulum-cell neoplasm, Type B	SJL	91	Virgin ♀ ♀	13.3
		High	Breeding, ♀ ♀, ♂ ♂	
Reticulum-cell neoplasm, Type A	C57BL	15	Breeding ♀ ♀	22.3
Ovarian tumor	C3HeB/De	37	Breeding ♀ ♀	21.5
		47	Virgin ♀ ♀	24.3
	C3HeB/Fe	64	Breeding ♀ ♀	After 19
		22	Virgin ♀ ♀	After 19
	RHI	60	Breeding ♀ ♀	After 17
		50	Virgin ♀ ♀	After 17
	CE	34	♀ ♀	After 20
Pituitary tumor	C57L	33	Breeding ♀ ♀	Old
	C57BR/cd	33	Breeding ♀ ♀	Old
Hemangioendothelioma	HR/De	24	♂ ♂ and ♀ ♀	22
Adrenal cortical tumor	CE	100	Gonadectomized ♀ ♀	After 6
		79	Gonadectomized ♂ ♂	After 7
Testicular teratoma	129	1	♂ ♂	Congenital
		82	(Male gonadal ridges transplanted to adult testes)	
Myoepithelioma	BALB/c	4		
	A	Similar		
Skin papilloma	HR/De	9	Hairless	22
Skin carcinoma	HE/De	3	Hairless	18
Subcutaneous sarcoma	C3H/J	3	♀ ♀	25
Harderian-gland tumor	C3H	1		20.7

From Murphy, E. D., Characteristic tumors, in *Biology of the Laboratory Mouse,* 2nd ed., Green, E. L., Ed., McGraw-Hill, New York, 1966, 523. With permission.

TABLE 4

Percentage of Incidence of Tumors of Some Long-lived Inbred Strains and Wild Mice[a]

	C3HeB/De				C3Hf/He		C57BL/He		DBA/2cBDe		HR/De			Wild Mice		
	♀♀	B♀♀	FB♀♀	♂♂	♀♀	B♀♀	♀♀	B♀♀	♀♀	B♀♀	♀♀	B♀♀	♂♂	♀♀	B♀♀	♂♂
Number of mice	99	155	82	21	100	471	471	314	76	51	48	63	52	72	99	54
Average age, months	23	19	19	21	20	19	19	21	22	21	22	16	21	24	27	21
Mammary carcinomas	4	55	74		2	40			3	6	4	30			6	
Type A		17	26			18									3	
Type B	4	23	28			19				6					2	
Type C									3							
Adeno-acanthoma		17	28			10										
Miscellaneous		5	4												1	
Mixed		<1	5													
Reticulum-cell neoplasms	2	3			3	3		25	20	27	12	10	8	11	12	5
Type A	2	<1					15	15	12	10	6	3	6	<1		1
Type B	2	2					11	11	8	18	6	6	2	11	12	5
Primary lung tumor	14	5	4	24	10	6		1	4	4	17	3	8	15	28	16
Hepatoma	59	30	38	90	17	25	25	<1	5		6	2	12	3	4	9
Ovarian tumors	47	37	29		8	6	6	<1			4	6		3	6	
Granulosa-cell tumor	20	23	12								2	5		3	6	
Tubular adenoma	25	14	15													
Luteoma	2	<1	1													
Papillary cystadenoma											2	2				

62   *Carcinogenesis Testing of Chemicals*

TABLE 4 (continued)

	C3HeB/De				C3Hf/He		C57BL/He		DBA/2cBDe		HR/De			Wild Mice		
	V♀♀	B♀♀	FB♀♀	♂♂	V♀♀	B♀♀	V♀♀	B♀♀	V♀♀	B♀♀	V♀♀	B♀♀	♂♂	V♀♀	B♀♀	♂♂
Hemangioendothelioma	2	5	1		2	3	3	2	12	16	19	14	29	3	8	
Lymphocytic neoplasm	1					<1		3	3	8	6	8	6		2	
Granulocytic leukemia									1	2						
Plasma-cell neoplasm			1						1							
Mast-cell neoplasm															1	
Subcutaneous sarcoma	7	2	1		3	3	3	3		4				1	2	
Osteogenic sarcoma					1		<1							1		
Uterine tumors																
Sarcoma	3				2						2					
Leiomyoma							<1		1			3				
Adenocarcinoma												2				
Endometrial sarcoma										2						
Adrenal cortical tumor				5					1		2					
Pheochromocytoma			1											3		
Harderian-gland tumor				5						2	2					2

TABLE 4 (continued)

	C3HeB/De				C3Hf/He		C57BL/He		DBA/2cBDe		HR/De			Wild Mice		
	V♀♀	B♀♀	FB♀♀	♂♂	V♀♀	B♀♀	V♀♀	B♀♀	V♀♀	B♀♀	V♀♀	B♀♀	♂♂	V♀♀	B♀♀	♂♂
Myoepithelioma			1									2				
Skin tumors																
Papilloma		<1			<1							2	4			
Squamous-cell carcinoma		<1			<1			<1				2	6			
Mammary-gland sarcoma												2				
Teratoma																2
Islet-cell tumor												2				
Granular myoblastoma					1											
Kidney carcinoma						<1										
Bladder papilloma					1											
Clitoral-gland tumor								<1								

From Murphy, E. D., Characteristic tumors, in *Biology of the Laboratory Mouse*, 2nd ed., Green, E. L., Ed., McGraw-Hill, New York, 1966, 524. With permission.

books, and they provide an introduction and a guide for further reading on spontaneous tumors of the mouse. The list is not intended to be complete or comprehensive. The Registry plans to issue lists of references in the future that will cover various aspects of pathology in the mouse, and will be glad to receive suggestions for revising and expanding the present and future lists.

C. Hamster

The Syrian golden hamster has frequently been used in routine experimental oncology, although much less frequently in routine tests for potential carcinogenicity of drugs. The Chinese hamster has been used to an even lesser extent. The majority of data on spontaneous tumors of hamsters refer to the Syrian strain (or inbred derivatives). Handler (1965) reviewed the literature and gives a detailed historic account of spontaneous neoplasia in the Syrian hamster.

The incidence of spontaneous tumors in this rodent is reported to be relatively low in most laboratories (Kirkman, 1962; Yabe, 1972; Fortner, 1957). Further references on spontaneous tumors in the Syrian hamster are listed below.

Its size, prolific breeding ability under laboratory conditions, and purported low incidence of spontaneous tumors suggest that the use of the hamster should be explored in routine carcinogenicity studies.

Further references to spontaneous tumors in the Syrian hamster are given below.

D. Dog

Although various breeds of dog, and particularly the beagle, have been widely used for routine toxicologic tests, this species has not been extensively used in assessing the carcinogenic potential of drugs. The comparatively long life span and the difficulty in housing and caring for an adequate number of animals are factors that contribute to this low frequency of use. Because of this infrequent use, most reports of spontaneous tumors in dogs have arisen in veterinary clinics or from cooperative reporting programs involving colleges of veterinary medicine and the National Cancer Institute. As such, the data do not represent the findings in a single laboratory. The environment under which the dogs had been housed is in some instances unknown, or at best unlike that in many industrial laboratories (pets or free-roaming animals as opposed to caged in laboratories), and this could influence tumor incidence. There is a paucity of published information on tumor incidence in dogs housed indoors in cages.

The degree of inbreeding must also be considered; many laboratories breed dogs for their own use, and consequent genetic changes could influence tumor incidence so that the data are not comparable to the general population of dogs.

Tumor incidence varies with breeds. Boxers, terriers, and the English bulldog, for instance, are reported to be predisposed to spontaneous tumors, whereas the beagle is considered to be less so.[D-14,15] Within the species, spontaneous tumors appear with greater frequency with advancing age (8th through 12th year).[D-16] From a survey of 202,277 animals, Priester and Mantel[D-17] reported the distribution of spontaneous tumor types (Table 5).

These authors also list relative risk of tumor

TABLE 5

Distribution of Spontaneous Tumors with Respect to Anatomic Sites in Dogs

Tumor type	% of total tumors (6,009)	References
Eye	3.6	4
Skin	28.1	12
Mammary	12.2	6
Bone	4.9	3, 7
Respiratory	3.9	
Hemic and Lymphatic	7.4	2, 11
Buccal	6.0	
Digestive	9.6	8
Urinary	1.2	
Genital	6.1	
Endocrine	2.9	5
Nervous	2.3	1
Other	12.0	

occurrence by breed. The noted references in Table 5 give information on the morphology and occurrence of spontaneous tumors in dogs. Ongoing long-term projects involving the beagle dog, such as the AEC studies being performed at the University of California at Davis (UCD472-111, Project 1-137), University of Utah, Lovelace Foundation, and at the Argonne National Laboratory, should give valuable information on incidence and morphology of spontaneous tumors in the beagle. References to these are also given below. Another group of long-term carcinogenic studies in dogs currently in progress are those being performed by various pharmaceutical manufacturers using the same protocol. It is hoped that results from these studies will add substantially to our knowledge of spontaneous tumors and related disease in caged dogs.

E. Monkey

In testing for carcinogenicity, the various animal species, and different strains within a species, vary in susceptibility to a particular agent. A particular type of animal may be selected in the hope that information gleaned from the model will have bearing on the agent's effects in man. Non-human primates are closest to man phylogenetically and are thus expected to provide the most accurate prediction of man's response.

In testing the potential of a chemical for carcinogenicity, the standard wild-caught monkey is rather unsatisfactory. Such animals are of unknown age and background. Frequently they are so debilitated from intercurrent disease that they die shortly after arrival in the laboratory. They may be used effectively for relatively short-term studies, but their unknown background precludes establishment of age-matched controls. The wide range of disorders incurred in the wild or in transit to the laboratory (Tauraso, 1973) makes it very difficult to match experimental and control groups with regard to past history, especially regarding exposure to known carcinogens.

Fewer than 200 spontaneous tumors have been described in various species of non-human primates (O'Gara and Adamson, 1972). Most of the data are case reports from zoological gardens or small laboratory colonies. Neoplastic disease has been observed in the skeletal system, sex organs, skin and subcutaneous tissue, liver, pancreas, lungs, gut, kidney, adrenal, and lymphoid tissue. The number of individual cases within a particular species is far too small to allow any prediction of expected spontaneous incidence of a specific neoplasm.

The regional primate centers supported by the National Institutes of Health have accumulated in excess of 7,700 primates of 45 species, thus providing an accelerated rate of base-line data acquisition regarding spontaneous tumors. In spite of the paucity of information, it is possible, and occasionally desirable, to use non-human primates for carcinogenesis testing of new drugs. Just as former users of pound (wild-caught) dogs and cats have found it in their own best interest to use laboratory-reared, defined-status animals, so has the investigator employing primate models. It is now feasible to rear some macaques and new-world monkeys in the laboratory. Breeding colonies have been established, with reproductive efficiency reported at up to 80%. These animals are as defined as any other laboratory-reared outbred experimental animal. They are expected to remain in relatively short supply for the next few years, although several commercial ventures are becoming established.

The occurrence and etiology of spontaneous lymphomas in new-world monkeys is certainly one of the more exciting discoveries in primate oncology. At the New England Regional Primate Research Center, of three cases of spontaneous lymphoma in the owl monkey, two have yielded a Herpesvirus, *H. saimiri* (Hunt, in press). This agent has a reservoir host, the squirrel monkey, *Saimiri sciureus,* and can be easily isolated from kidney, whole blood, and peripheral lymphocyte cultures. If marmosets (*Saguinus* sp.) or owl monkeys are experimentally inoculated with *H. saimiri*, 80% develop malignant lymphoma and 10% a lethal reticuloproliferative disease. Most deaths occur between 20 and 50 days after inoculation (Hunt, and Melendez, 1971).

A second oncogenic Herpesvirus, *H. ateles,* was isolated from a non-inoculated control marmoset that died of malignant lymphoma after being housed with *ateles*-inoculated animals. In this instance, the presumed transfer of agent was between individual susceptible hosts.

The full range of reservoir and susceptible hosts of these two oncogenic agents remains to be established. The current status is given in Table 6. The implications for carcinogenesis testing in the indicated species are that "spontaneous" tumors can be induced in susceptible hosts intentionally

TABLE 6

Lymphoma Viruses of Monkeys: Oncogenic Range in Animals

Animals		Herpesviruses	
Species	Common name	ateles	sai-miri
Saimiri sciureus	Squirrel monkey	–	–[a]
Aotus trivirgatus	Owl monkey	±	+
Saguinus oedipus	Cotton-top marmoset	+	+
Saguinus nigricollis	White-lipped marmoset	nt	+
Callithrix jacchus	Tufted-eared marmoset	nt	+
Cebus albifrons	Cinnamon ringtail	nt	+
Ateles geoffroyi	Spider monkey	–[a]	+
Macaca mulatta	Rhesus monkey	nt	–
Papio hamadryas	Baboon	nt	–
Cereopithecus aethiops	African green monkey	nt	±
Macaca aretoides	Stumptailed monkey	nt·	–
Pan troglodytes	Chimpanzee	nt	–
Oryctolagus cuniculis	New Zealand white rabbit	–	+

[a]Natural reservoir. – = nonsusceptible; + = susceptible; nt = not tested; ± = lymphoreticuloproliferative disorder.

Taken from *Fed. Proc.,* 31, 1648, 1972. With permission.

by artificial inoculation, or accidentally by errors in management that lead to caging reservoir and susceptible hosts together. (It is interesting to note that Herpesviruses have been indirectly associated with oncogenicity in the case of EB virus in Burkitt's lymphoma, nasopharyngeal carcinoma, infectious mononucleosis, and Hodgkin's lymphoma in man.)

In summary, the relative paucity of information on most aspects of the non-human primate, especially spontaneous tumors, plus the inadequate numbers of well-defined, laboratory-reared animals is expected to severely restrict the use of non-human primates in tests for carcinogenicity. In spite of these significant impediments, primate models are being used.

IV. CONCLUSIONS AND RECOMMENDATION

The spontaneous appearance of neoplasia in laboratory animals is an important consideration in the selection of a species for tests for the carcinogenicity potential of new drugs. It is only through comparison of differences of tumor occurrence between treated and control groups of

[‡]The use of inbred strains δ or G hybrids is recommended.

animals that adequate assessment of carcinogenic potential can be made. Of the many animal species available for use, the overwhelming majority of data on spontaneous tumors is in rodent species. Of these, the broadest data base exists for the rat and the mouse. There is, however, a great deal of variability in spontaneous-tumor occurrence between the rat and the mouse, as well as between strains of either species. An investigator should familarize himself with available data before selecting a strain for carcinogenicty tests.[‡] Consideration should be given to the time and location of tumor appearance as well as to the incidence of tumor occurrence. The capability of spontaneous (as well as of induced) tumors for metastasizing should also be considered. The investigator should also be aware of the susceptibility of the rat and the mouse to endocrine or endocrine-dependent tumors. This fact should be taken into consideration when selecting a strain for carcinogenicity evaluation of a drug with known endocrine pharmacologic effects. The relative practicality of housing sufficient numbers of rodents for their life span eases the complex task of collecting data on spontaneous tumors in these species. It is recommended that each laboratory determine the spontaneous-tumor incidence in the strain of animals used in their own particular facility, taking into consideration the following factors:

1. Characterization of the environment;
2. Characterization of the diet and its components;
3. Concomitantly occurring non-neoplastic diseases;
4. Source of animals.

In contrast to the rat and the mouse, less is known on spontaneous tumors of other animal species studied over their life span. The scientific value of carcinogenicity studies in other species, i.e., dogs or primates, is obvious; however, their relatively long life span makes their use on a routine basis impractical for testing in carcinogenicity. Nonetheless, for those specific instances in which a dog or a primate would be the species of choice for a carcinogenicity experiment, adequate data on spontaneous-tumor incidence are lacking. It is recommended that further research be conducted in the area of spontaneous-tumor development in various breeds of dogs and in non-human primates. It is further recommended that spontaneous-tumor incidence in species not specifically covered here (guinea pig, rabbit, gerbil, cat and swine) should be studied.

REFERENCES

A. Rat

1. **Tannenbaum, A.,** in *The Physiopathology of Cancer,* 2nd ed., Homburger, F., Ed., Harper and Row, New York, 1959, 517.
2. **Hadidian, Z., Fredrickson, T. N., Weisburger, E. K., and Weisburger, J. H.,** *Toxicol. Appl. Pharmacol.,* 8, 343, 1966.
3. **Snell, K. C.,** in *The Pathology of Laboratory Animals,* Ribelin, W. E. and McCoy, J. R., Eds., Charles C Thomas, Springfield, 1965, 241.
4. **Shubik, P., Saffiotti, U., Lijinsky, W., Pietra, G., Rappaport, H., Toth, B., Raha, C. R., Tomatis, L., Feldman, R., and Ramahi, H.,** *Toxicol. Appl. Pharmacol.,* 4 (Suppl. 4), 62, 1962.
5. **Davis, R. K., Stevenson, G. T., and Busch, K. A.,** *Cancer Res.,* 16, 194, 1956.
6. **Durbin, P. W., Williams, M. H., Jeung, N., and Arnold, J. S.,** *Cancer Res.,* 26, 400, 1966.

B. Mouse

1. **Dunn, T. B.,** Spontaneous lesions of mice, in *The Pathology of Laboratory Animals,* Ribelin, W. E. and McCoy, J. R., Eds., Charles C Thomas, Springfield, 1965, 303.
2. **Staats, J.,** for the Committee on Standardized Nomenclature for Mice, Standardized nomenclature for inbred strains of mice: Fifth listing, *Cancer Res.,* 32, 1609, 1972.
3. **Dunn, T. B. and Andervont, H. B.,** Histology of some neoplasms and non-neoplastic lesions found in wild mice maintained under laboratory conditions, *J. Natl. Cancer Inst.,* 31, 873, 1963.
4. **Dunn, T. B.,** Normal and pathologic anatomy of the reticular tissue in laboratory mice, with a classification and discussion of neoplasms, *J. Natl. Cancer Inst.,* 14, 1281, 1954.
5. **Dunn, T. B. and Deringer, M. K.,** Reticulum cell neoplasm, Type B, or the "Hodgkin's-like lesion" of the mouse, *J. Natl. Cancer Inst.,* 40, 771, 1968.
6. **Heston, W. E., Vlahakis, G., and Deringer, M. K.,** High incidence of spontaneous hepatomas and the increase of this incidence with urethane in C3H, C3Hf, and C3He male mice, *J. Natl. Cancer Inst.,* 24, 425, 1960.
7. **Hilberg, A. W.,** Morphologic variations in an osteogenic sarcoma of the mouse when transplanted to the kidney, *J. Natl. Cancer Inst.,* 16, 951, 1956.
8. **Dunn, T. B.,** Plasma cell neoplasms beginning in the ileocecal area in strain C3H mice, *J. Natl. Cancer Inst.,* 19, 371, 1957.
9. **Rask-Nielsen, R. and Gormsen, H.,** On the occurrence of plasma-cell leukemia in various strains of mice, *J. Natl. Cancer Inst.,* 16, 1137, 1956.
10. **Dunn, T. B. and Potter, M.,** A transplantable mast cell neoplasm in the mouse, *J. Natl. Cancer Inst.,* 18, 587, 1957.
11. **Rask-Nielsen, R. and Christensen, H. E.,** Studies on a transplantable mastocytoma in mice. I. Origin and general morphology, *J. Natl. Cancer Inst.,* 30, 743, 1963.
12. **Graffi, A.,** Chloroleukemia of mice, *Ann. N.Y. Acad. Sci.,* 68, 540, 1957.
13. **Dunn, T. B., Heston, W. E., and Deringer, M. K.,** Subcutaneous fibrosarcomas in strains C3H and C57BL female mice, and F$_1$ and backcross hybrids of these strains, *J. Natl. Cancer Inst.,* 17, 639, 1956.
14. **Russell, E. S. and Fekete, E.,** Analysis of W-series pleiotropism in the mouse: Effect of W^{v}W^v substitution on definitive germ cells and on ovarian tumorigenesis, *J. Natl. Cancer Inst.,* 21, 365, 1958.
15. **Munoz, N. and Dunn, T. B.,** Primary and transplanted endometrial adenocarcinoma in mice, *J. Natl. Cancer Inst.,* 41, 1155, 1968.

16. Dunn, T. B., Normal and pathologic anatomy of the adrenal gland of the mouse, including neoplasms, *J. Natl. Cancer Inst.,* 44, 1323, 1970.
17. Furth, J. and Clifton, K. H., Experimental pituitary tumors and the role of pituitary hormones in tumorigenesis of the breast and thyroid, *Cancer,* 10, 842, 1957.
18. Upton, A. C., Kimball, A. W., Furth, J., Christenberry, K. W., and Benedict, W. H., Some delayed effects of atom-bomb radiation in mice, *Cancer Res.,* 20 (8, Pt. 2), 1, 1960.
19. Stevens, L. C., Studies on transplantable testicular teratomas of strain 129 mice, *J. Natl. Cancer Inst.,* 20, 1257, 1958.
20. Dunn, T. B., Cancer of the uterine cervix in mice fed a liquid diet containing an antifertility drug, *J. Natl. Cancer Inst.,* 43, 671, 1969.
21. Slye, M., Holmes, H., and Wells, H. G., The comparative pathology of cancer of the thyroid, with report of primary spontaneous tumors of the thyroid in mice and in a rat, *J. Cancer Res.,* 10, 175, 1926.
22. Morris, H. P., The experimental development and metabolism of thyroid gland tumors, *Adv. Cancer Res.,* 3, 51, 1955.
23. Jones, E. E. and Woodward, L. J., Spontaneous adrenal medullary tumors in hybrid mice, *J. Natl. Cancer Inst.,* 15, 449, 1954.
24. Fekete, E. and Ferrigno, M. A., Studies on transplantable teratoma of the mouse, *Cancer Res.,* 12, 438, 1952.
25. Nettleship, A., Study of a spontaneous mouse rhabdomyosarcoma, *J. Natl. Cancer Inst.,* 3, 563, 1943.

C. Hamster
1. Handler, A., Spontaneous lesions of the hamster, in *Pathology of Laboratory Animals,* Ribelin, W. E. and McCoy, J. R., Eds., Charles C Thomas, Springfield, 1965, 210.
2. Kirkman, H., *Stanford Med. Bull.,* 20, 163, 1962.
3. Yabe, Y., Kataoka, N., and Koyama, H., *Gann,* 63, 329, 1972.
4. Fortner, J. G., *Cancer,* 10, 1153, 1957.

Additional References
5. Ashbel, R., *Nature,* 155, 607, 1945.
6. Chesterman, F. C. and Pomerance, A., *Br. J. Cancer,* 19, 802, 1965.
7. Fortner, J. G., *Arch. Surg.,* 77, 627, 1958.
8. Fortner, J. G., *Cancer Res.,* 21, 1491, 1961.
9. Fortner, J. G. and Allen, A. C., *Cancer Res.,* 18, 98, 1958.
10. Fortner, J. G., George, P. A., and Sternberg, S. S., *Endocrinology,* 66, 364, 1960.
11. Fortner, J. G., Mahy, A. G., and Cotran, R. S., *Cancer Res. Cancer Chemother. Screening Data,* X21(6), 199, 1961.
12. Fortner, J. G., Mahy, A. G., and Schrodt, G. R., *Cancer Res. Cancer Chemother. Screening Data,* X21(6), 161, 1961.
13. Friedell, G. H., Oatman, B. W., and Sherman, J. D., *Transplant. Bull.,* 7, 97, 1960.
14. Handler, A. H. and Cohn, J., *Proc. Am. Assoc. Cancer Res.,* 3(2), 116, 1960.
15. Kirkman, H., *Prog. Exp. Tumor Res.,* 16, 201, 1972.
16. Kirkman, H. and Robbins, M., *Proc. Am. Assoc. Cancer Res.,* 2(1), 28, 1955.
17. Toth, B., *Cancer Res.,* 27, 1430, 1967.
18. Webber, M. M., Jones, M. G., and Connolly, J. G., *Invest. Urol.,* 5, 348, 1968.
19. Chen, H. C., in *Progress in Experimental Tumor Research,* Vol. 16, Pathology of the Syrian Hamster, Homburger, R., Ed., Phiebig, White Plains, N.Y., 1972, 637.

D. Dog
1. Adams, C. W. and Slaughter, L. J., *Pathol. Vet.,* 7, 498, 1970.
2. Alroy, J., *Vet. Pathol.,* 9(2), 90, 1972.
3. Brodey, R. S., *J. Am. Vet. Med. Assoc.,* 159(10), 1242, 1971.
4. Barnett, K. C., *J. Small Anim. Pract.,* 13, 315, 1972.
5. Conroy, J. D. and Breen, P. T., *Vet. Med. Small Anim. Clin.,* 67, 297, 1972.
6. Cotchin, E., *J. Comp. Pathol. Ther.,* 68, 1, 1958.
7. Hamilton, J. M. and Kight, D., *Vet. Rec.,* 92, 41, 1973.
8. Murray, M., Robinson, P. B., McKeating, F. J., Baker, G. J., and Lauder, I. M., *Vet. Rec.,* 91(20), 474, 1972.
9. Norris, W. P., *J. Am. Vet. Med. Assoc.,* 152, 1085, 1968.
10. Richards, M. A. and Mawdesley-Thomas, L. E., *J. Pathol.,* 98, 283, 1969.
11. Squire, R. A., *Natl. Cancer Inst. Monogr.,* 32, 97, 1969.
12. Talerman, A. and Gwynn, R., *J. Pathol.,* 101, 62, 1970.
13. Zakarian, B., Naghshineh, R., and Sanjar, M., *J. Small Anim. Pract.,* 13, 249, 1972.
14. Lombard, C., *Cancerologie Comparée Cancer Spontané. Cancer Experimental,* Doin, Paris, 1962.
15. Zaldivar, R., *J. Am. Vet. Med. Assoc.,* 151(9), 1186, 1967.

16. Howell, J. and Ishmael, J. J., *Small Anim. Pract.,* 11, 793, 1970.
17. Priester, W. A. and Mantel, N., *J. Natl. Cancer Inst.,* 47, 1333, 1971.
18. Jones, T. and Gilmore, C. E., Pathologic Findings in Aged Dogs and Cats, NAS Publication No. 1591.

AEC Project
19. Andersen, A. C., Annual Progress Report No. 14. UCD 472-111, U.S.A.E.C., University of California School of Veterinary Medicine, Radiobiology Project, April 1965.
20. Andersen, A. C. et al., *Exp. Gerontol.,* 1, 193, 1965.
21. Wolf, H. G., Della Rosa, R. J., and Andersen, A. C., *Lab. Anim. Care,* 16, 309, 1966.
22. Guttman, P. H. and Andersen, A. C., *Radiat. Res.,* 35, 45, 1968.
23. Andersen, A. C. and Rosenblatt, C. S., *Radiat. Res.,* 39, 177, 1969.
24. Fristz, T. E. et al., ANL-7409, U.S.A.E.C., Argonne National Laboratories, 1967, 283.

E. Monkey
1. Tauraso, N. M., Review of recent epizootics in non-human primate colonies and their relation to man, *Lab. Anim. Sci.,* 23, 201, 1973.
2. O'Gara, R. W. and Adamson, R. H., Spontaneous and induced neoplasms in non-human primates, in *Pathology of Simian Primates,* Part 1, Fiennes, R. N., Ed., Phiebig, White Plains, N.Y., 1972, 190.
3. Hunt, R. D. et al., *J. Infect. Dis.,* in press.
4. Hunt, R. and Melendez, L., *J. Natl. Cancer Inst.,* 49, 261, 1971.

SECTION 12
REPORT OF DISCUSSION GROUP NO. 8[a]
CRITERIA FOR TUMOR DIAGNOSIS AND CLASSIFICATION OF MALIGNANCY

Melvin Reuber

The ultimate criteria for malignancy are the spread of carcinomas or sarcomas by invasion in the organ of origin, extension into nearby organs, or metastases to other organs by blood stream lymphatics. Since such data are not always available, and may not become available, other means of evaluation must be provided. The most reliable method is subcutaneous transplantation of a fragment of tissue measuring 3 X 6 mm to an untreated isologous host, using *inbred animals* of the same strain. The tissue for transplantation should be carefully selected. The host should be four weeks of age and of the same sex as the donor. The tumor transplants should not only survive, but should grow more than one transplant generation and kill the animal by reaching a large size or by metastasizing to other organs. Transplantation studies make possible a correlation of the biologic behavior with the histological pattern of tumors. Furthermore, the results can be used for interpretation of tumors in random-bred animals.

Malignant tumors can be divided into (1) ductal or adenocarcinomas and carcinomas derived from other epithelial cells, and (2) sarcomas. There are various degrees of differentiation, and this degree is reflected in the histological diagnosis. It also varies somewhat in the various organs. Vague terms, such as hepatoma, cholangioma, adenomatosis, and reticular-cell neoplasm, should be discarded; they should be replaced by more specific terms, such as hepatocellular carcinoma, cholangiocellular carcinoma, and malignant lymphoma, reticulum-cell type. Benign tumors are adenomas. A malignant tumor should both grossly and microscopically compress the adjacent tissue and not be microscopic in size. The entire tumor should be made up of malignant cells. There is disagreement, but a lesion with atypical cells or with focal malignant change should probably be included in a category of its own rather than under malignant tumors.

TUMORS OF THE LIVER

The morphologic and biologic correlation of tumors of the liver has been studied in detail in rats and mice.[1-11] Transplantation of tumors has provided a means of describing the histological criteria for malignant tumors of the liver. Carcinomas can be divided into hepatocellular carcinomas and cholangiocarcinomas. Both types can be subdivided into two categories: well differentiated and poorly differentiated.

Hepatocellular Carcinomas

These carcinomas arise from parenchymal cells; they often retain the vesicular nuclei, and sometimes the eosinophilic cytoplasm. Poorly differentiated carcinomas grow in sheets and generally can be fairly easily recognized. The criteria are those for anaplasia: (1) size and shape of nuclei and cells; (2) presence of abnormal mitotic figures; (3) cytoplasm is usually basophilic, but can be darkly eosinophilic; and (4) nuclei are vesicular, with prominent nucleoli.

Well-differentiated hepatocellular carcinomas are more difficult to recognize and often are incorrectly diagnosed. Histologically these carcinomas retain many of the characteristics of normal liver cells. Criteria for malignancy need not be those of anaplasia, but are the following: (1) formation of cords, two or several layers in thickness, with canaliculi, and prominent sinusoids with lining cells; (2) cytoplasm is usually darkly eosinophilic, but can be basophilic; (3) cytoplasm is either decreased or increased in amount; (4) nuclei are vesicular, with prominent nucleoli, and (5) absence of double nucleated cells or mitotic figures. Formation of cords with canaliculi can often be the most helpful indication of well-differentiated carcinomas. Occasional carcinomas may be made up predominantly of canaliculi and can contain bile casts. Glycogen is rarely, if ever, present.

---

[a]The full text of the Report of Discussion Group No. 8 is reproduced here as it was presented at the Conference. However, the Group felt that sufficient time had been devoted only to the discussion of liver tumors and that its Final Report should be limited to the introduction, discussion of tumors of the liver, and recommendations. Inclusion of material referring to other types of tumors should be regarded as providing background information only.

Cholangiocarcinomas

These carcinomas retain many of the characteristics of bile duct cells, i.e., columnar cells with lightly basophilic cytoplasm and oval nuclei. Well-differentiated cholangiocarcinomas are fairly easy to recognize. They have the following criteria: (1) formation of ducts, sometimes containing mucin in the cytoplasm or lumens; (2) cytoplasm is lightly basophilic; (3) "desmoplastic" background of fibrous connective tissue; and (4) nuclei are oval, with inconspicuous nucleoli; and (5) lack of mitotic figures.

Poorly differentiated cholangiocarcinomas grow in sheets and have (1) oval cells and nuclei with some mitoses; (2) lightly basophilic cytoplasm; and (3) fibrous connective-tissue stroma. They appear to be attempting to form ducts.

Undifferentiated Carcinomas

Undifferentiated carcinomas grow in sheets. They are more anaplastic than poorly differentiated carcinomas and have (1) great variation in size and shape of nuclei and cells; (2) basophilic cytoplasm; (3) frequent abnormal mitoses; and (4) nucleoli that are prominent, and often more than one.

Sarcomas

The most frequent sarcomas of the liver are hemangioendothelial sarcomas. Well-differentiated hemangiosarcomas retain many of the characteristics of endothelial cells. They are made up of (1) spindle-shaped cells with spindle-shaped nuclei; and (2) vascular spaces filled with red blood cells. Less-differentiated sarcomas are easily diagnosed because of their anaplastic characteristics. However, they also form, to some degree, vascular spaces.

The liver must be examined carefully for hemangioendothelial sarcomas. These can be small and can grossly resemble an area of recent hemorrhage. Sometimes the cellular areas are also obscured by the red blood cells on the histologic section.

Leiomyosarcomas, fibrosarcomas, and reticulum-cell sarcomas are rarely observed in the liver.

Other Lesions of the Liver

It is recognized that hyperplastic nodules, adenomas, and cysts will be present in the livers of animals with carcinomas. It is not the purpose of this group to discuss the subject at this time.

TUMORS OF THE LUNG

The lesions of the lung referred to as pulmonary adenomas are often adenocarcinomas. These grow in sheets, and the usual criteria of anaplasia used for liver and other organs can be used for poorly differentiated or undifferentiated carcinomas of the lung. They are fairly easy to recognize.

The well-differentiated adenocarcinomas usually form glands. The cells should have (1) lightly basophilic cytoplasm; (2) oval or round nuclei; and (3) lack of mitotic figures. It would appear that the presence of papillary structures and of mucin probably indicates malignancy.

Hemangioendothelial sarcomas can be primary in the lungs, but most often they are metastatic from the liver.

Squamous-cell carcinomas were discussed briefly at this time. The diagnosis of this cell type does not appear to be as complicated as that for adenocarcinomas.

LYMPHOMAS AND LEUKEMIAS

Lesions of lymph nodes or nodules and infiltrates in organs should be diagnosed as lymphoma. Leukemia refers to diffuse involvement of spleen, bone marrow, and in some cases to lymph nodes and increased numbers of malignant cells in the blood stream. Most lymphomas and leukemias replace the normal structure of lymph nodes and/or the spleen and bone marrow. The sternum and the vertebrae are good bones to study for the diagnosis of leukemia. Smears of blood are also helpful in the diagnosis of leukemias.

The present classification of the lymphomas and leukemias in rodents is unnecessarily complicated and difficult to understand. Diagnoses, such as type A or type B reticular neoplasms, are often vague and have no real value.

The lymphomas should be classified according to the dominant cell types as: (1) lymphocytic; (2) lymphoblastic; or (3) reticulum-cell.

Leukemias should be classified as (1) myelogenous or granulocytic; (2) lymphocytic; (3) lymphoblastic; or (4) erythroblastic. The predominant cell type for lymphomas and leukemias rarely may be plasma cells.

Occasionally, the diagnosis might be stem cell, or a type that is so undifferentiated that the cell cannot be identified. In such cases, the less-differentiated or undifferentiated cells may be associated with mature cells, which could be a clue to their type. Granulocytic leukemia should be distinguished from myeloid metaplasia.

These cell types are illustrated in histology and hematology books and are not described here.

TUMORS OF THE MAMMARY GLAND

The present classification of carcinomas of the mammary gland in rodents is confusing and complicated. These tumors should be studied and classified as ductal or lobular carcinomas, with the various degrees of differentiation. It appears that the presence or absence of metastases may be related to the location of the primary tumor.

It is felt that the criteria for poorly differentiated or undifferentiated carcinomas of the mammary gland are similar to those for other organs. However, members of the committee did not feel qualified at this time to list the criteria for malignancy of well-differentiated adeno-carcinomas. There is a need to distinguish the latter from fibroadenomas and adenomas.

RECOMMENDATIONS

The members of this discussion group feel that the criteria for malignancy need to be more clearly defined for each organ. Additional research should be carried out in order to establish such criteria. This research should include histogenesis and transplantation studies. Emphasis should be placed on the value of electron microscopy in the diagnosis of malignancy.

There is a need for the preparation and publication of monographs (similar to the Armed Forces Institute of Pathology Tumor Atlases) dealing with each of the organs, classifying, describing, and illustrating the characteristics of malignant tumors. The illustrations definitely should be in color. Each monograph discussing an organ should contain material relevant to all rodents. This could be best accomplished by a task force that would work on, evaluate, and approve each monograph.

The area that causes the most problems is that of lesions in which there are focal, atypical or malignant cells. Should this be considered as a malignant tumor? This "gray area" needs to be clarified. This may be a problem for the statisticians.

REFERENCES

1. **Reuber, M. D. and Firminger, H. I.,** Morphologic and biologic correlation of liver lesions obtained in hepatic carcinogenesis in AxC rats given a 0.025 percent N,2-fluorenyldiacetamide, *J. Natl. Cancer Inst.,* 31, 1407, 1963.
2. **Reuber, M. D.,** Development of preneoplastic and neoplastic lesions of the liver in male rats ingesting 0.025 percent N,2-fluorenyldiacetamide, *J. Natl. Cancer Inst.,* 34, 697, 1965.
3. **Reuber, M. D.,** Histopathology of transplantable hepatic carcinomas induced by chemical carcinogens in rats, *Gann Monogr.,* 1, 43, 1966.
4. **Reuber, M. D. and Glover, E. L.,** Hyperplastic and early neoplastic lesions of the liver in Buffalo stain rats of various ages given subcutaneous carbon tetrachloride, *J. Natl. Cancer Inst.,* 38, 891, 1967.
5. **Reuber, M. D. and Odashima, S.,** Further studies on the transplantation of lesions in hepatic carcinogenesis in rats given 0.025 percent 2-(diacetoamino)-fluorene, *Gann,* 58, 513, 1967.
6. **Reuber, M. D.,** Histogenesis of cholangiofibrosis and well-differentiated cholangiocarcinoma in Syrian hamsters given 2-acetamidofluorene or 2-dineactoamidofluorene, *Gann,* 59, 239, 1968.
7. **Reuber, M. D. and Lee, C. W.,** Effect of age and sex on hepatic lesions in Buffalo strain rats ingesting diethylnitrosamine, *J. Natl. Cancer Inst.,* 41, 1133, 1968.
8. **Reuber, M. D.,** Hyperplastic and early neoplastic lesions of the liver in rats of varying ages with dietary-induced cirrhosis, *Tumori,* 55, 79, 1969.
9. **Reuber, M. D. and Glover, E. L.,** Cirrhosis and carcinoma of the liver in male rats given subcutaneous carbon tetrachloride, *J. Natl. Cancer Inst.,* 44, 419, 1970.
10. **Reuber, M. D.,** Morphologic and biologic correlation of hyperplastic and neoplastic hepatic lesions occurring "spontaneously" in C3HxY hybrid mice, *Br. J. Cancer,* 25, 538, 1971.
11. **Herrold, K. McD.,** Histogenesis of malignant liver tumors induced by dimethylnitrosamine: an experimental study in Syrian hamsters, *J. Natl. Cancer Inst.,* 39, 1099, 1967.

SECTION 13
REPORT OF DISCUSSION GROUP NO. 10
METABOLIC ACTIVATION AS A FACTOR IN CARCINOGENIC RESPONSE

Daniel Nebert

Chemical carcinogenesis results from delivery of the appropriate ultimate carcinogen — at an appropriate rate — to the appropriate cellular target, so that a permanent modification in cellular homeostasis appears (Figure 1). Any pathways of detoxification or excretion of the xenobiotic will affect the rate at which the proximal or ultimate carcinogen is formed. Also, there are certain compounds that do not require metabolic activation. A pathway that is a detoxification pathway for one drug might be an activation pathway for

another compound. Any pathway of deactivation or excretion and the stability or the reactivity of the intermediate will influence the rate at which the target is attacked. A form of deactivation for one intermediate may potentiate the intermediate of another drug to interact at an increased rate with the target. In all likelihood, the "target" represents cellular information molecules, such as nucleic acids. Any lethal effects causing cell death or any pathways leading to repair of the target will modify the rate at which sublethal permanent

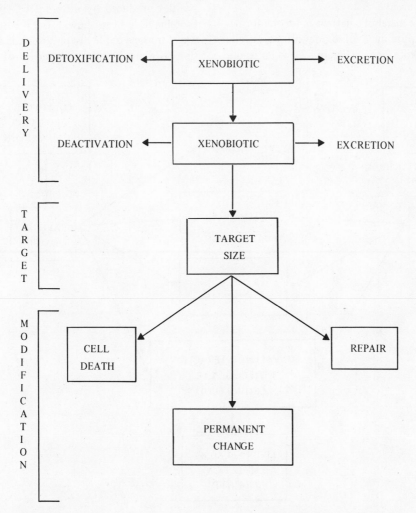

FIGURE 1. General scheme by which xenobiotic-initiated carcinogenesis may occur.

changes in cellular homeostasis occur. For example, all cocarcinogens examined have the capacity to block DNA repair. Further, all mutagenic acridine dyes tested inhibit DNA repair, whereas all nonmutagenic acridine analogs tested do not inhibit DNA repair. The initiation and the promotion of tumorigenesis therefore depend on a delicate balance between the nine possible pathways by which a xenobiotic travels. This delicate balance probably differs among species of animals, among strains of the same species, among tissues from the same animal, and among cells in the same tissue. Moreover, this delicate balance is no doubt influenced by the age of the animal, by nutritional and hormonal differences, by such periodic factors as circadian rhythmicity, mitotic index, and cell cycle, and by exposure of the animal to other pharmacologically or toxicologically active environmental agents.

The possible metabolic pathways for the formation and disappearance of oxides of polycyclic aromatic hydrocarbons (Figure 2) is a more specific example of this general scheme. Although these pathways were discussed in greatest detail by our group, it became apparent that the metabolic fate of polycyclic hydrocarbons is extremely complex and poorly understood. There are clearly two spectrally distinct CO-binding hemoproteins — cytochrome P-450 and cytochrome P-448 — which are associated with the enzyme-active site for epoxidation of the parent molecules. There is growing evidence that both cytochrome P-450 and cytochrome P-448 are composed of subsets of different enzymically active hemoproteins, so that two or three (or perhaps ten or twenty) specific CO-binding cytochromes exist. Different hemoproteins may metabolize a given xenobiotic at different positions, producing arene oxides of varying degrees of reactivity and in varying quantities. Several examples of dissimilar metabolite profiles produced by different CO-binding hemoproteins have been shown. The predominant pathway for arene oxide disappearance is via isomerization to phenols; other properties of these oxides

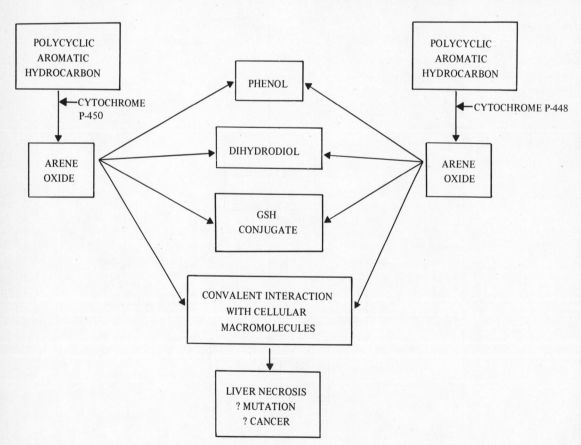

FIGURE 2. Possible metabolic pathways for the formation and disappearance of oxides of polycyclic aromatic hydrocarbons.

include rearrangement to other arene oxides, rearrangement to reactive ketones, and solvolysis and other nucleophilic reactions. In addition, there are enzymes that react with the arene oxides: epoxide hydrases, which cause dihydrodiol formation, and epoxide-glutathione transferases, which form mercapturic acid precursors. Once again, several hydrases and several transferases have been characterized, and it is possible that there exist ten, twenty, or more of these types of enzymes with differing substrate specificities. Lastly, arene oxides may bind covalently to specific target molecules. In all likelihood, a large quantity of nonspecific covalent binding in the cell also occurs. Any of these factors influencing the level and lifetimes of arene oxides may affect the reaction of the ultimate carcinogen with the cellular target. Compounds with electron-withdrawing groups lead to arene oxides that are more stable and thus potentially more dangerous. At present, however, no firm statements can be made concerning the number of enzymes involved or the specificities of these enzymes in activating molecules to the ultimate carcinogen.

It should be emphasized that compounds may become activated by pathways other than through the intervention of cytochromes P-450 and P-448. In general, ultimate carcinogenic derivatives are usually electrophilic reactants, e.g., alkylating agents and potential alkylating agents that yield electrophilic reactants in the nonenzymic alkylation of nucleic acids and proteins in vitro at pH 7. N-Hydroxylation has been strongly implicated in the formation of proximal carcinogenic derivatives, and this reaction can be either P-450-mediated or non-P-450-mediated, depending on the compound and the particular cell or tissue. Hydroxylation and carbonium ion formation of methyl groups of the polycyclic aromatic hydrocarbons, sulfuric acid esterification, acetic acid esterification, O-glucuronidation, acetylation, and free-radical formation are yet other non-P-450-mediated reactions implicated in the metabolic activation of compounds to form the proximal or ultimate carcinogen.

What, then, are the recommended areas for future study in this field? The first area (Table 1) is that of delivery. We need to understand drug metabolism at a mechanistic level to the end that this approach may give insight into the nature of carcinogenic initiation and perhaps insight into methods for reversing such metabolic activation. This area involves the tedious identification of proximal and ultimate carcinogens for each compound in a specific tissue or in a specific cell population (such as tissue culture), the solubilization and characterization of all enzymes involved in the activation and deactivation pathways, and

TABLE 1

Recommended Areas for Future Study

A. Delivery

    1. Identification of intermediates and metabolites
    2. Solubilization and characterization of all enzymes involved
    3. Selective enzyme induction or inhibition
    4. Correlation of genetic differences in cancer susceptibility to genetic differences in enzyme levels

B. Target Site

    1. Specific interaction versus nonspecific binding
    2. Metabolic activation in liver and target interaction in nonhepatic tissue?

C. Modification of Cellular Homeostasis

    1. Inhibition of normal cellular repair mechanisms
    2. Specific genetic alteration

D. Development of New Drugs

    1. Quantitative index of carcinogenicity
    2. Antioxidants as a form of treatment?

ultimately the extrapolation of such findings in vitro and in cell culture to the intact animal in which a carcinogenic index for a given compound might be predicted. Manipulation of these metabolic pathways — by experimental modifications, such as selective enzyme induction or inhibition, or by correlation of genetic differences in cancer susceptibility to genetic differences in enzyme levels — may bypass some of the exhaustive biochemical characterizations of every enzyme.

The second area is that of understanding the interaction between the carcinogenic agent and informational target molecules. In general, electrophiles will bind to nucleophilic molecules, such as nucleic acids. The obvious difficulty in this area is to separate the specific target interaction from the much larger quantities of nonspecific binding to cellular macromolecules. The possibility was raised that relatively stable reactive proximal carcinogens — activated in the liver, but then circulated throughout the animal — may interact with target molecules in nonhepatic tissues.

The third area is that of defining cellular homeostasis and understanding how xenobiotics can sublethally modify homeostasis so that a cancerous cell can evolve. This is particularly relevant with respect to cocarcinogens that can interfere with normal cellular repair mechanisms. An agent should be particularly carcinogenic if it both modifies the target site and prevents repair of the target.

The fourth area is that of drug development, the theme of this conference. Can one predict the potential carcinogenicity of a drug by some quantitative simple index? Covalent binding appears to be a general reflection of a compound's metabolic reactivity with cellular macromolecules. One might, therefore, consider modifying a given drug by the insertion of certain chemical groups, which would not alter the pharmacological activity, but would markedly change the covalent reactivity of the drug. Whereas antioxidants may decrease the interaction of nucleophiles with the important target, this form of "treatment" for decreasing the incidence of chemically induced carcinogenesis may be a two-edged sword. For example, in Figure 1 a lethal event might be modified by antioxidants in such a way that a sublethal but permanent change in homeostasis occurs.

Although the ultimate solution to chemical carcinogenesis must be understood at the molecular level, there is continuing need to study these processes at the level of animal models. At this point in time, it seems essential to realize that carcinogenesis is a complex process, and our present knowledge would *not* suggest that a single approach will be adequate.

SECTION 14
HISTORICAL EVOLUTION OF SHORT-TERM TESTS FOR CARCINOGENICITY

David B. Clayson

The need for short-term tests is nearly as old as the serious study of chemical carcinogenesis. Kennaway's classic search between 1920 and 1930 for the factors in coal tar that are responsible for the induction of carcinomata of human and mouse skin was hampered by the need for lengthy painting tests in mice at each stage in the fractionation. The large quantities of material required for these tests further impeded progress. Hieger[29] observed that the active fractions had two characteristic bands in their fluorescence spectrum, which he identified with the benz(a) anthracene structure (Figure 1). This knowledge led rapidly to the preparation of the first synthetic carcinogenic polycyclic hydrocarbon, dibenz(a,h)-anthracene, and to the first isolation of benzo(a) pyrene from coal tar.[9,10]

A parameter such as a common fluorescence spectrum is essentially a means of identifying a partial molecular structure that is believed to confer carcinogenic properties on the whole molecule. It is, in fact, one way of deriving the probable carcinogenicity of a substance from its chemical structure. As our knowledge of carcinogens has increased, the possibilities of predicting this property from the structure of a molecule have also increased. If a chemical possesses any of the characteristics shown in Table 1, the probability that it will induce tumors is substantially increased. This is, in fact, the first, and obvious, screen that all new drugs (and other environmental chemicals) should be put through. The factors to be considered with drugs are the following: (1) Does the potential drug bear a formal structural relationship to any known carcinogen? (2) What are the consequences if a potentially carcinogenic chemical is not allowed to enter the pharmacopoeia; that is to say, can the drug be used to treat a hitherto incurable condition? Unfortunately, our knowledge of the molecular parameters responsible for the induction of cancer is still too limited to rely only on this approach and other methods are required.

CRITERIA FOR SHORT-TERM TESTS

It is necessary to define the criteria to which a short-term screening test should adhere before it is possible to judge which of the available tests is likely to be useful. In my opinion the following aspects are essential:

1. The limits within which the tests are operative should be closely defined. Is the test applicable to all classes of carcinogens, e.g., asbestos or metals?

2. The tests should incorporate some specific attribute of the carcinogen or the carcinogenic process; tests that involve the chance association of a physical, chemical, or biological property in a limited series of carcinogenic situations are unlikely to hold over a wide range of agents. For example, although there was a theoretical basis for the possible importance of charge-transfer in polycyclic aromatic hydrocarbon carcinogenesis, the suggestion that the complexing of carcinogens with molecules such as iodine or acridine was applicable to all polycyclic aromatic carcinogens[55] failed when subjected to an extensive test.[14] For this reason, no attempt will be made in this paper

AROMATIC HYDROCARBONS WITH COMMON FLUORESCENCE SPECTRUM

Benz(a)anthracene

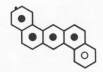

Dibenz (a,h) anthracene

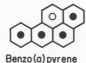

Benzo(a)pyrene

FIGURE 1. Aromatic hydrocarbons with a common fluorescence spectrum. The realization that coal-tar fractions exhibited the fluorescence spectrum of benz(a)-anthracene led to the isolation of benzo(a)-pyrene and the synthesis of benz(a,h)anthracene and other polycyclic hydrocarbons. (Taken from Hieger, I., *Biochem. J.*, 24, 505, 1930. With permission.)

TABLE 1

Main Classes of Compounds Containing Chemical Carcinogens

Group	Notes and examples
Alkylating agents	Mustards, epoxides, ethylene-imines, strained-ring lactones, alkanesulfonates, nitrosamides
Polycyclic aromatic hydrocarbons	Ring N-, O-, S-substituted derivatives
Aromatic amines	Nitro compounds, nitroso compounds, heterocyclic derivatives
N-Nitroso compounds	Aliphatic rather than aromatic
Hydrazides and hydrazines	
Triazides	
Azo compounds	Aminoazo compounds
Chlorocarbons	
Hormones	Estrogens, especially diethylstilbestrol and estrone
Metals and other inorganics	Asbestos, nickel, etc.
Radiochemicals	Bone-seeking isotopes

to list the many tests that have been discarded because it was discovered that the assumptions on which they were based were not applicable to all the carcinogens under consideration.

3. It should be demonstrable that compounds with known carcinogenic properties should be positive within the limits of the test, and negative compounds negative. If the test is required for preliminary screening, a small proportion of false negative or positive results may be acceptable. If a final test is visualized, *no* false negative results are acceptable.

4. For use in the drug industry, in particular, a test should be economical to carry out. The pharmaceutical industry has an exceedingly high rate of wastage between the synthesis of new compounds by the organic chemist and the final marketing of a new drug. Because long-term tests for carcinogenesis take some years to complete, much expensive development work is often completed before the result of the carcinogenicity tests is known. Thus, if a substance induces tumors, it is probable that this effort will be wasted with the discarding of the substance. An economical test could be applied to a range of potential drugs early in their development, thus eliminating most carcinogens at an early stage.

Short-term tests may be used in two ways. They may be needed to trace a carcinogen in a complex environmental situation, as was the case with coal tar, or they may be required to screen large numbers of new drugs and other chemicals. The environmental problem is the easier of the two and has in the past been investigated mainly by in vivo tests, while in vitro methods that are now being developed offer greater possibilities for the investigation of, for example, ranges of new drugs. This difference in approach arises because in the search for environmental factors the tissue in which the tumors arise is known, whereas with new drugs any tissue or tissues may be affected.

IN VIVO TESTS

Short-term in vivo tests for skin carcinogens have been examined most extensively, but some pointers to pathologically useful phenomena in other tissues are known.

Skin — The lengthy and costly work on the

bladder lumen. Thus, although this in vivo indication of carcinogenicity has been successful in the comparatively few examples to which it has been applied, the different biological processes that lead to the development of bladder hyperplasias seem not to augur well, so far, for its wider application.

Liver — Magee and Barnes[36] noticed that dimethylnitrosamine induced centrilobular necrosis in rat liver during subacute toxicity testing. This led them to carry out full carcinogenicity tests on this compound, with results that are too familiar to need repetition. Recently Nishie et al.[39] returned to this typical property of liver carcinogens in rodents and suggested that, if studied in mice, it provides a useful screening test for carcinogenic nitrosamines. The quantity of nitrosamine sufficient for this type of test (30 mg/kg body weight/day) is excessive. As much information will be obtained from the structure of the nitrosamine as from this test. Also, nitrosamines induce tumors in tissues other than liver, e.g., in the esophagus.

Compressed Carcinogenicity Tests

Compressed or shortened carcinogenicity tests cover those examples in which enhanced tumor induction is assayed against a relatively high natural tumor incidence, as with lung adenomas in A-strain mice or hepatomas in male C3H mice. They usually last 6 to 12 months. Hypothetical age-versus-incidence curves (Figure 3) demonstrate the reason for my anxiety lest these tests replace full-length tests. By terminating the experiment at the appropriate time, it is possible to get approximately equal enhancement in tumor yields from experimental group 1 and either control group 1, 2, or 3 (Figure 3). Yet the significance one would place on the results of these experiments is very different. For this reason, one must judge the enhanced yields of liver tumors induced by the neonatal administration of a variety of substances, or the use of pulmonary adenomas in anything but well-defined research situations, with caution. Tumor induction is species-, strain-, and tissue-specific, and the work of Tannenbaum[56] on the effects of dietary modification in both these tumors shows a further element of doubt in the interpretation of such results in terms of the carcinogenicity of the test materials. Counting individual pulmonary adenomas is considered a satisfactory solution to the difficulties that arise in mouse lung, but it needs further study if it is to be used as a general rather than as a research-orientated screening test.

Other compressed carcinogenicity tests may arise from current research effort. Transplacental carcinogenesis and various forms of initiation and promotion systems offer opportunities for the rapid induction of tumors. However, these appear to me to be liable to the same difficulties in interpretation as full-length carcinogenicity tests and probably will be more restricted in view of the

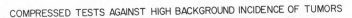

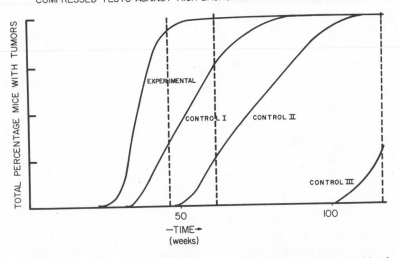

FIGURE 3. Carcinogenicity tests carried out against high background yields of tumors may be as statistically significant as those carried out against low background yields, but they engender less confidence.

identification of the carcinogens present in catalytically cracked oil, a process that was introduced during World War II to increase the yield of high-octane fuels,[51] led Smith[50] to suggest the sebaceous gland suppression test for the rapid detection of oil fractions containing mouse skin carcinogens. This method was based on original observations by Simpson and Cramer[48] and depends on the "disappearance" of the sebaceous glands in mouse skin shortly after painting with a solution of a carcinogen. Solvents such as acetone tend to increase the cellularity of the sebaceous glands. The method can be quantitated by counting the number of active sebaceous glands in a standard area of mouse skin. Recently the technique has been modified. The sebaceous glands contain a high proportion of the non-specific esterase in the skin, and this may be demonstrated by histochemical staining. Healey et al.[25,26] therefore stained frozen sections of mouse skin for this enzyme and measured the level of staining in the Quantimet analyzing computer. The staining was inversely correlated with the skin carcinogenicity of a series of fractions of a tobacco condensate, which had previously been assayed by conventional painting on mouse skin to determine whether tumors developed. Nevertheless, the specificity of the test is in doubt. Skin carcinogens that do not lead to suppression of the sebaceous glands include: 7,9-dimethylbenz(c)acridine, beta-propiolactone, butadienediepoxide, and the initiator of mouse skin carcinogenesis, urethane. On the other hand, chemicals that have not been proved to be mouse skin carcinogens, such as the inhibitor of mitotic division of cells in metaphase, colchicine, have proved to be active.[4,25] Perhaps a greater degree of attention to the quantity of test substance to be administered, and to the time at which observations are made, would help to eliminate these discrepancies.

Two other short-term tests for skin carcinogens have been described: the hyperplasia test, and the formazan deposition test. In the hyperplasia test, the suspected carcinogen is painted on the mouse skin in acetone, or occasionally benzene, solution on days 1, 4, and 7 of the test, and the skin is examined histologically for hyperplasia.[24,49] The formazan deposition test is a measure of mitochondrial oxidizing function of the skin. Iversen and Evensen[30] measured the amount of formazan produced by incubating a piece of isolated tissue, from carcinogen-treated skin, with a solution of

2,3,5-triphenyltetrazolium chloride. Both meth[ods] have not been extensively examined for t[heir] specificity; however, the published results do [not] offer a substantially greater degree of specific[ity] than the sebaceous gland suppression test.

Pathological Observation from Subacute Toxicit[y] Tests

Subacute toxicity tests may, in some tissues, give an indication of the possible oncogenicity of the substance under observation.

Bladder — Some of our observations on the induction of bladder epithelial hyperplasia during the early period of treatment (2 to 10 weeks) suggested that test substances inducing this hyperplasia might be bladder carcinogens.[7] This suggestion was used predictively on two occasions in mice and once in rats (Figure 2), namely with 3-aminodibenzofuran,[6] dibutylnitrosamine,[59] and 2(n-butyloxycarbonylmethylene)thiazolid-4-one.[1] Wood,[58] as a result of her comparative studies of the influence of the sex of mice on the hyperplasiogenic and carcinogenic effects of 2-acetyl-aminofluorene in the bladder, concluded that the correlation is not absolute. Levi et al.[33] showed that the hyperplasias induced by 2-acetylamino-fluorene and 4-ethylsulfonylnaphthalene-1-sulfonamide were, at the cellular level, of different types. 2-Acetylaminofluorene induced hyperplasia by a slow increase in cell number, whereas the sulfonamide induced a wave of cell destruction and regeneration that led to hyperplasia by over-compensative growth in the first days of treatment, and later this hyperplasia was maintained by reaction of the epithelium to the concretions of calcium and ammonium phosphate formed in the

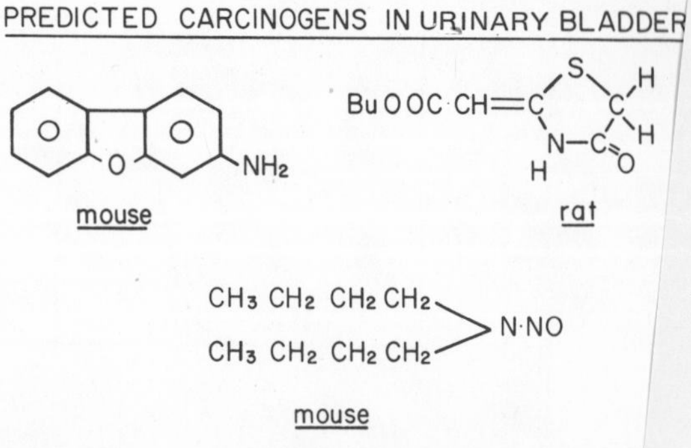

PREDICTED CARCINOGENS IN URINARY BLADDER

FIGURE 2. The early development of epith[elial] hyperplasia of the bladder epithelium led to the disc[overy] of the illustrated molecules in the species listed.

different ability of different chemicals to pass the placental barrier or to initiate specific tissues.

Summary

Short-term tests carried out in vivo are tissue-dependent and usually rely on non-cancerous or premalignant changes, such as hyperplasias, alterations in the structure of the affected tissue, or other such toxic phenomena. They have great value when a carcinogenic factor is to be isolated from a mixture that is known to contain carcinogens, but are of little use for screening large numbers of drugs of unknown activity and tissue-specificity. Even if a short-term biological test were to be developed for every tissue, the amount of skilled labor involved in operating such a scheme would make it as impracticable and uneconomical as the long-term test.

IN VITRO TESTS

In my view, in vitro short-term carcinogenicity tests should mimic part or all of the carcinogenic process in the living animal. The chemical induction of cancer now appears to be divisible into three phases (Figure 4). In the first phase, the agent is metabolically activated to a highly reactive positive ion[38] or, possibly, a radical ion.[2] In the second phase, this unstable intermediate reacts with cellular constituents, of which DNA, RNA, and protein have been most extensively examined, and gives rise to cells with altered properties. DNA repair represents the reverse of this process. In the third phase, cells that have been suitably altered by interaction with the carcinogen develop into a tumor within the environment provided by the host organism. Metabolic activation is now suggested to be the main determinant leading to species, strain, and dietary influences in carcinogenesis.

In certain groups of compounds, such as the biological alkylating agents, e.g., mustards or strained-ring lactones, the carcinogens are sufficiently reactive not to need further activation by the host, although detoxication mechanisms may still play a part in determining tumor yield and localization. Again, it is possible that, with certain compounds, interaction with cellular constituents to form covalent macromolecule—carcinogen bonding may not be essential. If this is the case, cells that have malignant potential through exposure to background environmental oncogens, such as viruses or traces of chemical carcinogens, may be stimulated to form tumors. Examples of this type possibly include tumors of certain endocrine or endocrine-responsive tissues after prolonged and massive exposure to hormones, especially estrogens.

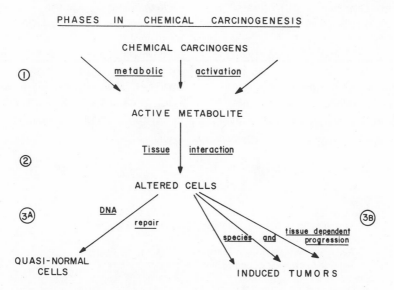

FIGURE 4. Carcinogenesis can be considered as a multiphase phenomenon. Phase 1 is the metabolic activation of the carcinogen; Phase 2 is the interaction of the activated carcinogen with the genome; Phase 3B represents the progression of the altered cells to a tumor, while Phase 3A demonstrates the possibility that DNA repair processes may lead to quasi-normal cells.

I am convinced that short-term in vitro tests need to be carried out on human as well as on animal tissues where they can be obtained without detriment to the patient. New short-term screening tests should make use of both human and animal tissues to avoid depriving mankind of new drugs. For example, our present aspirations to develop a carcinogen-free pharmacopoeia would have eliminated the effective and valuable antituberculous agent isoniazid on the possibly unfounded suspicion of being a carcinogen in man.

Laboratory models for full, long-term carcinogenicity tests are, at best, compromises forced on the experimentalist · by the entirely proper necessity to adhere to civilized codes of ethical conduct, which prohibit such tests in man.

The first clue to the design of short-term in vitro tests came from Dustin,[11] who reported that a range of chemicals shared some of the properties of radiation (Table 2). Of these properties, mutagenesis seemed to be the most appropriate for the design of suitable short-term tests, especially as one of the intellectually satisfying explanations of cancer is the somatic-mutation theory. However, Burdette,[5] in 1955, pointed out that the relation between carcinogenesis and mutation was most inexact. Potent carcinogens, such as the polycyclic hydrocarbons or the aromatic amines, were, at best, very weak mutagens, whereas weak carcinogens, such as certain nitrogen mustards, were potent mutagens. Over the past 18 years, the position has been greatly changed in light of the discovery of metabolic activation. It now seems likely that the majority of the activated carcinogens will be demonstrated to be mutagenic and that a considerable proportion of mutagens, if administered in an effective manner, may be carcinogenic.[37] Mutagenicity induced in mono-

cellular organisms is therefore capable of development into a screening test for carcinogenicity.

The Host-mediated Assay

The host-mediated assay (Figure 5) was introduced by Gabridge and Legator[20] to demonstrate substances that become mutagenic on metabolic activation. The method consisted of injecting intraperitoneally a suspension of monocellular organisms, such as strains of *Salmonella typhimurium* or *Neurospora*, and coincidentally administering the test substance to mice. The organisms were isolated from the peritoneum after a suitable interval, and the number of mutants formed, in comparison to those induced in a standard in vitro test, was determined. It is thus possible to determine whether the test substance is mutagenic with or without metabolic activation or whether the host detoxifies the substance. Legator and Malling[32] have recently reviewed the use of the method, and Table 3 is adapted from their text.

Garner et al.[23] demonstrated that the method could be used completely in vitro by incubating the test substance and the monocellular organisms with microsomes and the necessary cofactors. Two parameters could be measured: the increase in toxicity of the microsomally activated carcinogen (aflatoxin) to the organisms, and the mutation rates. In more recent work, using strains of *Escherichia coli*, Garner has established that mutant microorganisms lacking the ability to repair UV-radiation-induced damage to DNA are most susceptible to the toxic action of aflatoxin. Furthermore, when microsomes were incubated with ^{14}C-labeled aflatoxin in vitro, binding to DNA, RNA and protein was similar to that found in vivo.[21,22] There appear to be considerable

TABLE 2

Radiation-like Effects

1. Cytotoxicity
   Vesicant action, hemoconcentration, diarrhea, and leukopenia
   Bone-marrow changes
   Reduction of circulating leukocytes
   Damage to sperm cells and precursors
2. Chromosome aberrations
3. Mutagenicity
4. Enzyme inhibition
5. Therapy of malignant disease
6. Carcinogenesis
7. Bleaching of hair

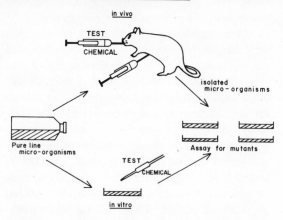

FIGURE 5. The technique of host-mediated assay involves the comparison of the mutagenic power of a chemical when tested in vitro and when tested in the peritoneum of the rodent after oral administration. It thus gives a measure of in vivo activation and detoxication of the compound.

pitfalls in this approach, because hamster liver, which has not been satisfactorily shown to be susceptible to the carcinogenic action of aflatoxin B in vivo, is the source of the most effective microsomes that have been examined in vitro. The difficulty probably arises because in Garner's work, to the present time, only the mixed-function oxidases have been activated by the addition of the necessary cofactors. In vitro use of the host-mediated assay is limited by the tissue from which the microsomes are obtained and by the cofactors chosen by the investigator. It is thus likely to be a research tool in the immediate future.

Carcinogenesis in vitro

The earliest attempts to induce cancer-like behavior in cells growing in culture were made by Earle, Sanford, and their collaborators.[12,13,45,46] Their efforts were frustrated because both their control and 3-methylcholanthrene-treated cultures developed malignant change after long but variable periods in culture. The changed cells were, however, genuinely tumorous and gave rise to sarcomas when implanted into mice of the inbred strain from which the original cultures were derived. The changes in culture that lead to tumor-producing cells, known as transformation, are seldom found in untreated cells maintained for relatively short periods in culture.

Freeman and Huebner[16] have recently called

TABLE 3

Summary of Initial Results and Host-mediated Assay Results with *Salmonella typhimurium* Strain G-46

Compound	In vitro	Host-mediated assay
1. 2-Aminopurine nitrate	+	−
2. Caffeine	−	−
3. Mitomycin C	−	−
4. Chloramphenicol	−	−
5. Streptozotocin	+	+
6. Neocarzinostatin	−	−
7. N-Methyl-N'-nitro-N-nitrosoguanidine	+	+
8. Hydroxylamine	−	−
9. Dimethylnitrosamine	−	+
10. Cycasin	−	+
11. Methylazoxymethanol	+	+
12. Bromouracil	+	−

Taken from Legator, M. S. and Malling, H. V., in *Chemical Mutagens: Principles and Methods for Their Detection*, Vol. 2, Hollaender, A., Ed., Plenum Press, New York, 1971, 569. With permission.

for the strict definition of malignant transformation; it should be used only if the altered cells have been shown to produce tumors on reimplantation into suitable host animals and to be isolatable as a pure cell line. The other changes in culture are referred to as morphological transformation and include the following:

1. Loss of contact inhibition, which is the normal state leading to untransformed cells forming a confluent culture.
2. Crisscross development and piling up.
3. Alterations in the shape of the cell or of any of its components.
4. Loss of adherence of the cell to the surface on which it is growing.

Berwald and Sachs[3] and Heidelberger and his associates[27,28,44] were the first to succeed in inducing malignant chemical transformation of mammalian cells in vitro. Berwald and Sachs added polycyclic hydrocarbons at levels ranging between 10 and 0.005 μg per ml of medium for periods ranging from 3 to 144 hours to freshly cultured hamster embryo cells. After 78 to 98 days, and after many passages, there was evidence of morphological transformation, which was shown to be malignant by implantation into hamsters and by observing the development of sarcomas in a considerable proportion of the hamsters. Control cultures and those treated with pyrene, chrysene, and 8-methylbenz(*a*)anthracene, which are not considered to be carcinogenic, failed to produce tumors under these conditions, whereas the carcinogens 10-methylbenz(*a*)anthracene, 7,12-dimethylbenz(*a*)anthracene, 3-methylbenz(*a*)anthracene, 3-methylcholanthrene, and benzo(*a*)pyrene did so. Similar results were obtained using cells from SWI mice.

Heidelberger's system was more complex. It consisted of treating fragments of C3H mouse prostatic tissue in culture with a polycyclic hydrocarbon and subsequently developing a series of cell lines from the dispersed organ culture. Cell lines from untreated organ cultures invariably died out, whereas those from polycyclic hydrocarbons persisted and underwent malignant transformation.

The difficulties with these approaches are threefold. First, the cells used must be able to activate the carcinogen; fibroblasts have the ability to activate polycyclic hydrocarbons, but, as far as I am aware, they do not carry the N-hydroxylases needed to activate aromatic amines. Second, mice and hamsters are often known to carry oncogenic viruses, and it is possible that the action of the chemical in vitro is activation of a latent oncogenic virus; this may or may not be true in vivo. Third, these techniques are time-consuming and sufficiently complicated not to be attractive for routine short-term tests.

A variation in the technique for carcinogenesis in vitro has arisen from the observations of Freeman and his associates,[19] who showed that treatment of rat embryo cells with murine leukemia virus followed by diethylnitrosamine led to morphological transformation. Attempts to grow the altered cells in animals failed to produce tumors. Transformation did not occur if either the virus or the chemical was used alone. The author suggested that the difficulty in demonstrating malignant transformation was due to the resistance of rats to highly antigenic tumors. That is to say, routine use of the technique was handicapped by both non-carcinogen- and active-carcinogen-treated cells failing to induce tumors on implantation.

Further work on the use of this test has been published; these cover a sufficient range of chemicals to make it clear that it is being considered as a short-term test for carcinogenicity. Virus and 3-methylcholanthrene or 7,12-dimethylbenz(*a*)anthracene gave morphological transforma-tion;[17,41] virus and (−)-*trans*-Δ^9-tetrahydrocannabinol induced malignant transformation;[43] virus was much more effective with city smog than with benzo(*a*)pyrene in inducing morphological transformation;[18] virus and cigarette smoke also gave rise to transformation. Again there are three difficulties in accepting this technique as a basis for a short-term test without considerable extra study. First, there is the absence of a full complement of enzymes capable of metabolic activation. Second, there is the difficulty in establishing malignant transformation, which must be regarded as essential before a positive result can be accepted. Third, Price and his associates[42] believe that the transformations reflect the virus rather than the chemical. The chemical, therefore, may be the key to activating the virus; in other words, only a single property of the chemical is reflected in the test, whereas a different property or series of properties may be needed for the total induction of tumors by the chemical. Clearly, a great deal of further investigation is needed before this technique is used routinely.

Macromolecular Binding of Carcinogens and DNA Repair

Although much effort has gone into studies of carcinogen interaction with DNA, RNA, protein, lipids, and polysaccharides, no clear-cut differences have been found that might be exploited as short-term tests for carcinogens. For a variety of reasons, interaction with DNA appears to be primarily concerned in the carcinogenic process, but in the case of the methylating carcinogens, at least, not all of the methylated DNA may be involved in alteration of the genome. Effective methylation leading to mutation and probably carcinogenesis is limited to the formation of 6-O-methylguanine and other minor methylated bases while the major product, 7-methylguanine, is probably not of critical importance.[31,34,35,40]

DNA repair concerns the removal of various lesions in DNA induced by radiation or carcinogenic chemicals. It is slightly more promising as a short-term test than the induction of the chemical lesion itself. Patients with Xeroderma pigmentosum lack one of the enzymes concerned in DNA repair.[5,7] As a result, they are deficient in the ability to eliminate the thymine dimers induced by ultraviolet radiation, and exposure to sunlight leads to an increasing level of erythema, ulceration, and eventually tumors of the skin. Stich and

TABLE 4

Comparative Levels of DNA Repair Synthesis in Xeroderma Cells Exposed to Ultraviolet, 4NQO, N-Acetoxy-AAF and MNNG

Patient	Sex	Ultra-violet (1,000 ergs/mm^2)	4NQO (2 × 10^{-6}M, 90 min)	N-Acetoxy-AAF (5 × 10^{-5}M, 5 hr)	MNNG (2 × 10^{-4}M, 90 min)
XP$_{H1}$	F	9.8	10.3	10.2	103
XP$_{H2}$	M	12.1	13.1	16.0	103
XP$_E$	F	21.5	20.2	22.9	102
XP$_V$	F	36.0	33.6	29.1	105
XP$_K$	M	56.6	55.7	60.8	107
Control	M + F	100%	100%	100%	100%

Taken from Stich, H. F., San, R. H. C., Miller, J. A., and Miller, E. C., *Nat. New Biol.*, 238, 9, 1972. With permission.

his associates[52,53] have shown that certain chemical carcinogens, such as 4-nitroquinoline-N-oxide, lead to repair in the DNA of cultured human fibroblasts, but to a much smaller degree in fibroblasts from Xeroderma patients. Unfortunately, some carcinogens, such as N-methyl-N-nitroso-N'-nitroguanidine, induce damage in the DNA that *is* repaired in Xeroderma fibroblasts[52,53] (Table 4). Thus, the further use of this approach depends on recognizing the types of DNA damage induced by various types of carcinogens.

Tumor Progression

Tumor progression, namely the processes that take place in the developing tumor between the first application of chemical (in the present context) and the death of the tumor-bearing animal,[15] does not appear to offer a useful screening test, because most of the events occur in a random fashion and are not readily apparent until the tumor is recognizable. Attempts to show that inhibition of the immune process by chemical carcinogens is related to their carcinogenic potency were unsuccessful.[47]

Conclusions and Summary

Some of the most fascinating work now in progress on the mechanisms of chemical carcinogenesis justifies itself not only by its intrinsic interest, but because it may have the potential to suggest short-term tests for chemical carcinogens. I have stressed certain areas of historical development because I believe they have a future as well as a history.

To conclude, it appears that tests that are applicable to the isolation of carcinogenic factors in an environmental situation are unlikely to be applicable to the screening of series of substances of unknown carcinogenic activity. The testing of such series of compounds requires one or more economical tests that closely simulate one or more of the key stages of the carcinogenic process and, especially, human patterns of metabolic activation.

A short-term screening test that is acceptable to all regulatory authorities will probably not be developed for many years. It seems reasonable to expect, in the not-too-distant future, a series of screens by which the pharmaceutical industry and others will be able to eliminate a large proportion of the carcinogenic substances that are, at present, failed by. a long-term test after the majority of the costly pharmacological testing and development work has been finished.

REFERENCES

1. Alcock, S. J., Pre-neoplastic change in the urinary tract caused by a potential drug, in *Proceedings of the European Society for the Study of Drug Toxicity,* IX, p. 289, 1968.
2. Bartsch, H., Miller, J. A., and Miller, E. C., N-Acetoxy-N-acetylaminoarenes and nitrosoarenes. One electron non-enzymatic and enzymatic oxidation products of various carcinogenic aromatic acethydroxamic acids, *Biochim. Biophys. Acta,* 273, 40, 1972.

3. Berwald, Y. and Sachs, L., *In vitro* transformation of normal cells to tumor cells by carcinogenic hydrocarbons, *J. Natl. Cancer Inst.*, 35, 641, 1965.

4. Bock, F. G. and Mund, R., A survey of compounds for activity in the suppression of mouse sebaceous glands, *Cancer Res.*, 18, 887, 1958.

5. Burdette, W. J., The significance of mutation in relation to the origin of tumors: a review, *Cancer Res.*, 15, 201, 1955.

6. Clayson, D. B., Lawson, T. A., and Pringle, J. A. S., The carcinogenic action of 2-aminodiphenylene oxide and 4-aminodiphenyl on the bladder and liver of the C57 x IF mouse, *Br. J. Cancer*, 21, 755, 1967.

7. Clayson, D. B., Lawson, T. A., Santanta, S., and Bonser, G. M., Correlation between the chemical induction of hyperplasia and of malignancy in the bladder epithelium, *Br. J. Cancer*, 19, 297, 1965.

8. Cleaver, J. E., Defective repair replication of DNA in Xeroderma pigmentosum, *Nature*, 218, 652, 1968.

9. Cook, J. W., Hewett, C. L., and Hieger, I., The isolation of a cancer-producing hydrocarbon from coal tar, Parts I, II and III, *J. Chem. Soc.*, p. 395, 1933.

10. Cook, J. W., Hieger, I., Kennaway, E. L., and Mayneord, W. V., The production of cancer by pure hydrocarbons, Part I, *Proc. R. Soc. Ser. B*, 111, 455, 1932.

11. Dustin, P., Some new aspects of mitotic poisoning, *Nature*, 159, 794, 1947.

12. Earle, W. R., Production of malignancy *in vitro*. IV. The mouse fibroblast cultures and changes seen in the living cells, *J. Natl. Cancer Inst.*, 4, 165, 1943.

13. Earle, W. R. and Nettleship, A., Production of malignancy *in vitro*. V. Results of injections of cultures into mice, *J. Natl. Cancer Inst.*, 4, 213, 1943.

14. Epstein, S. S., Bulon, I., Koplan, J., Small, M., and Mantel, N., Charge-transfer complex formation, carcinogenicity and photodynamic activity in polycyclic compounds, *Nature*, 204, 750, 1964.

15. Foulds, L., *Neoplastic Development*, Academic Press, New York, 1969, 439.

16. Freeman, A. E. and Huebner, R. J., Guest editorial: Problems in interpretation of experimental evidence of cell transformation, *J. Natl. Cancer Inst.*, 50, 303, 1973.

17. Freeman, A. E., Kelloff, G. J., Gilden, R. V., Lane, W. T., Swain, A. P., and Huebner, R. J., Activation and isolation of hamster-specific C-type RNA viruses from tumors induced by cell cultures transformed by chemical carcinogens, *Proc. Natl. Acad. Sci. U.S.A.*, 68, 2386, 1971.

18. Freeman, A. E., Price, P. J., Bryan, R. J., Gordon, R. J., Gilden, R. V., Kelloff, G. J., and Huebner, R. J., Transformation of rat and hamster embryo cells by extracts of city smog, *Proc. Natl. Acad. Sci. U.S.A.*, 68, 445, 1971.

19. Freeman, A. E., Price, P. J., Igel, H. J., Young, J. C., Maryak, J. M., and Huebner, R. J., Morphological transformation of rat embryo cells induced by diethylnitrosamine and Murine Leukemia Viruses, *J. Natl. Cancer Inst.*, 44, 65, 1970.

20. Gabridge, M. G. and Legator, M. S., A host-mediated microbial assay for the detection of mutagenic compounds, *Proc. Soc. Exp. Biol. Med.*, 130, 831, 1969.

21. Garner, R. C., Microsome-dependent binding of aflatoxin B_1 to DNA, RNA, polyribonucleotides and protein *in vitro*, *Chem.-Biol. Interactions*, 6, 125, 1973.

22. Garner, R. C., personal communication, 1973.

23. Garner, R. C., Miller, E. C., and Miller, J. A., Liver microsomal metabolism of aflatoxin B_1 to a reactive derivative toxic to *Salmonella typhimurium* TA 1530, *Cancer Res.*, 32, 2058, 1972.

24. Guerin, M. and Cuzin, J., Tests cutanés chez la souris pour déterminer l'activité carcinogène des goudrons de fumée de cigarettes, *Bull. Assoc. Fr. Etud. Cancer*, 48, 112, 1961.

25. Healey, P., Mawdesley-Thomas, L. E., and Barry, D. H., Short-term test for evaluating potential carcinogenic activity of tobacco condensates, *Nature*, 228, 1006, 1970.

26. Healey, P., Mawdesley-Thomas, L. E., and Barry, D. H., The effect of some polycyclic hydrocarbons and tobacco condensates on non-specific esterase activity in sebaceous glands of mouse skin, *J. Pathol.*, 105, 147, 1971.

27. Heidelberger, C., Studies on the cellular and molecular mechanisms of hydrocarbon carcinogenesis, *Eur. J. Cancer*, 6, 161, 1970.

28. Heidelberger, C. and Iype, P. T., Malignant transformation *in vitro* by carcinogenic hydrocarbons, *Science*, 155, 214, 1967.

29. Hieger, I., LVIII. The spectra of cancer-producing tars and oils and of related substances, *Biochem. J.*, 24, 505, 1930.

30. Iversen, O. H. and Evensen, A., Experimental skin carcinogenesis in mice, *Acta Pathol. Microbiol. Scand. Suppl.*, 156, 1, 1962.

31. Lawley, P. D. and Thatcher, C. J., Methylation of deoxyribonucleic acid in cultured mammalian cells by N-methyl-N'-nitro-N-nitrosoguanidine. The influence of cellular thiol concentrations on the extent of methylation and the 6-oxygen atom of guanine as a site of methylation, *Biochem. J.*, 116, 693, 1970.

32. Legator, M. S. and Malling, H. V., The host—mediated assay, a practical procedure for evaluating potential mutagenic agents in mammals, in *Chemical Mutagens: Principles and Methods for Their Detection*, Vol. 2, Hollaender, A., Ed., Plenum Press, New York, 1971, 569.

33. **Levi, P. E., Knowles, J. C., Cowen, D. M., Wood, M., and Cooper, E. H.,** Disorganization of mouse bladder epithelium induced by 2-acetylaminofluorene and 4-ethylsulfonylnaphthalene-1-sulfonamide, *J. Natl. Cancer Inst.,* 46, 337, 1971.

34. **Loveless, A.,** Possible relevance of O-6 alkylation of deoxyguanosine to the mutagenicity and carcinogenicity of nitrosamines and nitrosamides, *Nature,* 223, 206, 1958.

35. **Gerchman, L. L. and Ludlum, D. B.** The properties of O^6-methylguanine in templates for RNA polymerase, *Proc. Am. Assoc. Cancer Res.,* 14, 13, 1973.

36. **Magee, P. N. and Barnes, J. M.,** The production of malignant primary hepatic tumours in the rat by feeding dimethylnitrosamine, *Br. J. Cancer,* 10, 114, 1956.

37. **Miller, E. C. and Miller, J. A.,** The mutagenicity of chemical carcinogens: Correlations, problems and interpretations, in *Chemical Mutagens: Principles and Methods for Their Detection,* Vol. 1, Hollaender, A., Ed., Plenum Press, New York, 1971, 83.

38. **Miller, J. A.,** Carcinogenesis by chemicals: an overview – G. H. A. Clowes Memorial Lecture, *Cancer Res.,* 30, 559, 1970.

39. **Nishie, K., Norred, W. P., Wasserman, A., and Keyl, A. C.,** Phototoxicity and differential hepatotoxicity as biological indicators of nitrosamine activity, *Toxicol. Appl. Pharmacol.,* 23, 680, 1972.

40. **O'Connor, P. J., Capps, M. J., Craig, A. W., Lawley, P. D., and Shah, S. A.,** Differences in the patterns of methylation in rat liver ribosomal ribonucleic acid after reaction *in vivo* with methyl methanesulphonate and N,N-dimethylnitrosamine, *Biochem. J.,* 129, 519, 1972.

41. **Price, P. J., Freeman, A. E., Lane, W. T., and Huebner, R. J.,** Morphological transformation of rat embryo cells by the combined action of 3-methylcholanthrene and Rauscher Leukemia Virus, *Nat. New Biol.,* 230, 144, 1971.

42. **Price, P. J., Suk, W. A., and Freeman, A. E.,** Type C RNA tumor viruses as determinants of chemical carcinogenesis: Effects of sequence of treatment, *Science,* 177, 1003, 1972.

43. **Price, P. J., Suk, W. A., Spahn, G. J., and Freeman, A. E.,** Transformation of Fischer Rat embryo cells by the combined action of Murine Leukemia virus and $(-)$-*trans*-Δ^9-tetrahydrocannabinol, *Proc. Soc. Exp. Biol. Med.,* 140, 454, 1972.

44. **Roller, M. R. and Heidelberger, C.,** Attempts to produce carcinogenesis in organ cultures of mouse prostate with polycyclic hydrocarbons, *Int. J. Cancer,* 2, 509, 1967.

45. **Sanford, K. K., Earle, W. R., Shelton, E., Schilling, E. L., Duchesne, E. M., Likely, G. D., and Becker, M. M.,** Production of malignancy *in vitro*. XII. Further transformations of fibroblasts to sarcomatous cells, *J. Natl. Cancer Inst.,* 11, 351, 1950.

46. **Sanford, K. K., Likely, G. D., and Earle, W. R.,** The development of variations in transplantability and morphology within a clone of mouse fibroblasts transformed to sarcoma-producing cells *in vitro, J. Natl. Cancer Inst.,* 15, 215, 1954.

47. **Scherf, H. R., Kruger, C., and Karsten, C.,** Untersuchungen an Ratten über immunosuppressive Eigenschaften von Cytostatica unter besonderer Berücksichtigung der carcinogenen Wirkung, *Arzneimittel-forschung,* 20, 1467, 1970.

48. **Simpson, W. L. and Cramer, W.,** Sebaceous glands and experimental skin carcinogenesis in mice, *Cancer Res.,* 3, 515, 1943.

49. **Skjaeggestad, O.,** Experimental epidermal hyperplasia in mice in relation to carcinogenesis, *Acta Pathol. Microbiol. Scand. Suppl.,* 169, 1, 1964.

50. **Smith, W. E.,** Sebaceous gland activity as a measure of the relative carcinogenicity of certain oils and tars, *Bull. N. Y. Acad. Med.,* 32, 77, 1956.

51. **Smith, W. E., Sunderland, D. A., and Sugiura, K.,** Experimental analysis of the carcinogenic activity of certain petroleum products, *Arch. Ind. Hyg.,* 4, 299, 1951.

52. **Stich, H. F. and San, R. H. C.,** DNA repair synthesis and survival of repair deficient human cells exposed to K region epoxides of benz(*a*)anthracene, *Proc. Soc. Exp. Biol. Med.,* 142, 155, 1973.

53. **Stich, H. F., San, R. H. C., and Kawazoe, Y.,** Increased sensitivity of Xeroderma pigmentosum cells to some chemical carcinogens and mutagens, *Mutat. Res.,* 17, 127, 1973.

54. **Stich, H. F., San, R. H. C., Miller, J. A., and Miller, E. C.,** Various levels of DNA repair synthesis in Xeroderma pigmentosum cells exposed to the carcinogens 'N-hydroxy and N-acetoxy-2-acetylaminofluorene, *Nat. New Biol.,* 238, 9, 1972.

55. **Szent-Gyorgi, A. and McLaughlin, J.,** Reaction of carcinogens with acridine, *Proc. Natl. Acad. Sci. U.S.A.,* 47, 1397, 1961.

56. **Tannenbaum, A. and Silverstone, H.,** Nutrition and the genesis of tumours, in *Cancer,* Vol. 1, Raven, R. W., Ed., Butterworth, London, 1957, 306.

57. **deWeerd-Kastelein, E. A., Keijzer, W., and Bootsma, D.,** Genetic heterogeneity of Xeroderma pigmentosum demonstrated by somatic cell hybridization, *Nat. New Biol.,* 238, 80, 1972.

58. **Wood, M.,** Factors influencing the induction of tumours of the urinary bladder and liver by 2-acetylaminofluorene in the mouse, *Eur. J. Cancer,* 5, 41, 1969.

59. **Wood, M., Flaks, A., and Clayson, D. B.,** The carcinogenic activity of dibutylnitrosamine in IFxC$_{57}$ mice, *Eur. J. Cancer,* 6, 433, 1970.

SECTION 15
SHORT-TERM TESTS FOR CARCINOGENESIS: TESTS INVOLVING INDUCTION OF NEOPLASIA

J. A. DiPaolo

If one considers the chronological development of carcinogenesis, it becomes obvious that chemicals have been implicated as human carcinogens for the last two centuries. I refer specifically to the observations of Hill,[1] who in 1761 described clinical symptoms similar to cancer in snuff users, and of Percival Pott,[2] who in 1775 reported a causal association between cancer and an environmental substance. The scrotal skin cancer in London chimney sweeps observed by Pott was concluded to be due to repeated deposits of coal soot for many years. This prompted the Danish chimney sweepers' guild to rule that its members have a daily bath, a ruling that was responsible for making scrotal skin cancer in chimney sweeps a relatively rare disease outside of England. Experimental confirmation of Pott' observation occurred in 1915; two Japanese investigators[3] reported that coal tar, when painted on the ears of a rabbit, resulted in skin cancer at the site of application in a few of the surviving rabbits. Subsequently, mice and rats were shown to be susceptible to tumor induction by various chemicals. Thus, the foundation for a major approach in chemical-carcinogenesis research was established: the induction of cancer in laboratory animals by substances presumed to be carcinogenic from epidemiologic data.

It is now estimated that 50 to 90% of all human cancers are due to chemical carcinogens.[4] It becomes obvious that the bioassay of compounds by routine in vivo testing is an insurmountable task, requiring time, proper facilities, and funds. Therefore, we have become interested in utilizing tissue culture for the development of in vitro models for screening environmental factors that are potential carcinogens to humans. Such in vitro model procedures, in comparison to established in vivo procedures, should be less costly in both time and money, require small samples of test chemicals for the test, yet be reliable, sensitive, and, very importantly, practical. Most important, the system should correlate well with clinical and in vivo carcinogenesis bioassays.

The use of mammalian cells in cultures is particularly appropriate, since it represents an extension of the in vivo experimental models. Furthermore, since it is possible to characterize the alterations produced by carcinogens in mammalian cells in a number of different ways, including the ability of the transformed cells to produce tumors, in vitro models utilizing mammalian cells become particularly relevant.[5-7] Any other type of short-term test for in vivo carcinogenesis assay must be considered an additional step further removed from relevancy if it does not involve potential tumor production. For example, although a carcinogen may be a mutagen, it is inappropriate to consider that a mutagen is necessarily a carcinogen. Therefore, until the relation between mutations and cancer is elucidated and the relevancy of specific mutations or any other tests in regard to cancer is determined, no end point other than potential tumor production can be considered.

It is my contention that mammalian cells in tissue-culture models that are reproducible and lend themselves advantageously to the methodologic aspects of the desired end point represent a useful and worthwhile model, regardless of whether or not the mammalian cell model has a cell-type counterpart of significance in the human population. Tissue-culture systems used in conjunction with chemicals that are potential carcinogens are most useful because of their genuine predictability of tumor production. Furthermore, if one adds quantitation in terms of number of cells that are transformed, it becomes possible to distinguish those changes resulting from the carcinogen that are pivotal to the production of the neoplastic transformation from those that are incidental by-products.[8]

Ordinarily, when one adds a chemical carcinogen to cells in culture, a certain amount of toxicity occurs. Obviously, the toxicity that is easiest to measure is cell death; lethality is proportional to the concentration of carcinogen used and the type of cells under consideration. In any event, one can consider that the population is made up of cells that are sensitive to the lethality caused by the chemical and those that are resistant to the lethality caused by the chemical. The best way to obtain a reflection of this phenomenon is by colony-counting. The morphological transformation is defined as a difference in growth pattern not seen in the control cultures. The transformation can also most easily be seen by examining discrete colonies. In systems that utilize fibroblasts, this alteration is characterized by a random crisscross pattern of cells not seen in the controls.[9] This alteration in population dynamics is permanent, since it is observed in both the original colonies that had been transformed and the cell lines that are derived from the transformed colonies. Our studies with classical carcinogens lead us to a number of conclusions. For a compound that requires activation, transformation is independent of toxicity, increases with concentration of carcinogen, and in terms of transformation there appears to be no safe dose.[10] Using statistical analysis of the transformation frequency, it has been possible to conclude that the distribution of the transformants is Poissonian and thus consistent with a one-hit hypothesis of carcinogenesis. If one recalculates transformation on the basis of the original number of cells that were at risk, thus assuming that toxicity did not occur, and plots transformation rate versus carcinogen concentration on a semi-log scale, a linear relationship with dose can be obtained. This finding, as well as lack of transformation in the absence of carcinogen, provides additional evidence that the transformation phenomenon is inductive in this system.

The question whether transformation is due to selection or induction and is direct or indirect (viral activation) may vary, depending on the type of system used. It is our position that with the Syrian hamster system, utilizing secondary or tertiary subcultures, transformation is both inductive and direct, since there is no indication of viral activation. First of all, the cells used have been tested for 18 different viruses, ranging from Reo virus, whose function is unknown, to oncogenic viruses, such as polyoma, SV-40, and the adenos, all of which transform hamster cells. The remaining test to be completed involves virus rescue. The addition of simian virus 40 or of the LLE 46 strain of adenovirus 7 to hamster cells previously transformed by 3-methylcholanthrene resulted in cells with additional transformation properties that are ordinarily associated with virus.[11] The hamster cells are negative for these as well as for the

hamster leukemia virus; also, Dr. R. C. Gallo recently demonstrated that cells are negative in terms of his test for reverse transcriptase.[11a] Thus, the evidence presented demonstrates that transformation with the hamster embryo system is direct and is not due to selectivity.

It has been our experience that, when permanently altered cells are isolated and grown to form a cell line, it is usually possible to inject these cells into animals and obtain tumors.[12,13] The evidence that the injected cells actually produce the tumors is based on a number of different factors. Probably the most important among these is that our analysis proves that the unique cross-band pattern of chromosomes of the tumor cells and that of the chromosomes of cells that were injected are ordinarily the same.[14] Thus, we have finite evidence that transformed cell lines do produce tumors. For the Syrian hamster system it has been determined that approximately 95% of the transformed cell lines produce tumors, and with the Balb/3T3 system 100% of the transformed cell lines produce tumors. It is my impression that people working on quantitative in vitro chemical carcinogenesis have probably returned more cells to animals and demonstrated more often that these cells are capable of producing tumors than any other group of oncologists or pharmacologists. The time is approaching, I feel, when the relation between the transformation observed in vitro and the subsequent tumor production will be of such a degree of positive correlation that this particular aspect of the assay will be taken for granted.

Thus far, the results obtained with known chemical carcinogens and non-carcinogens correlate very highly with the results that are obtained in vivo. The different number of transformants observed was related to the known carcinogenic potency of the compounds tested.[15] As new in vitro models for testing carcinogenicity of chemicals are developed, it will become necessary to test the validity of the models by testing some of the same compounds in vivo. This results in the dilemma as to which compounds should be tested: those that produced transformations, or those that did not. Obviously, there is a possibility of false positives and false negatives. From a theoretical point of view, one can accept a certain number of false positives, but, obviously, false negatives would be a much more serious situation. Therefore, depending on the importance of the drug and its analogues, it may be desirable to test both groups of compounds or just the group containing some of the compounds that have been negative in the tests. This, of course, would not be necessary after confidence is developed in the in vitro assays being used.

Obviously, cells in tissue culture, soon after being placed in culture, cannot be considered normal; there is evidence, however, that they are not transformed either, since controls remain flat and the cells usually do not produce tumors. In addition, they are not necessarily capable of carrying out all the metabolic functions that they were carrying out in vivo. As a consequence, we have found it necessary to alter the in vitro assay to take into consideration certain known carcinogens that were inactive when applied directly to cells, presumably because such compounds required conversion to active agents by enzymes unavailable in culture. This resulted in a variation that we have termed "host-mediated in vivo-in vitro combination bioassay."[16] In this system, one additional step has been added to our standard technique, namely, the chemical to be tested is injected intraperitoneally into a pregnant hamster 48 to 72 hours prior to removal of the fetus. Subsequently the cells are prepared in normal fashion, and the transformation is eventually scored as the frequency of transformed colonies.

Because of the difficulties involving chemical carcinogens that might present themselves in attempting to transform different types of cells, we have become interested in the combined actions of chemicals with viruses[17] or radiation[18] in the transformation of hamster cells. If hamster cells are pretreated with X-irradiation, cloned at varying intervals, and treated with chemical carcinogen, the transformation produced by chemical carcinogen increases on a per-cell and per-total-colony basis. The increase in transformation with increased carcinogen concentration was independent of concentration of carcinogen within the range used. No transformation was recognized among the colonies of cells that survived radiation-only treatment. In other studies it was possible to obtain quantitative data to show that, following pretreatment of hamster cells in vitro with carcinogenic polycyclic hydrocarbons, the frequency of transformation of SA 7 type was enhanced.

However, treatment of cells 5 hours after virus addition resulted in an inhibition of transformation. There is indication that the stimulation of viral transformation resulted from a direct effect of the chemicals upon the cells, increasing their sensitivity to transformation.

The assays that I am recommending cannot be considered routine and should be used in conjunction with other biological studies. In the past, the interaction of chemical substances and biological systems have proven to be intriguing, exciting, and rewarding, as well as highly productive of information directly applicable to important problems in pharmacology. Opportunities to use these bioassays in conjunction with problems of a fundamental nature will contribute information on the pharmacological aspects of drug therapy at the cell level as well as on the biology of cancer, and thus ensure that the screening program does not become sterile.

In vitro models will make it possible to determine the nature of the cell—target interaction, the chemical nature of the ultimate carcinogen, the degree to which any agent acts alone, be it viral, chemical, or radiation, and the extent to which one agent interacts with another agent from the same or from a different category of carcinogens. In the past, particularly when the etiological effect has been weak or dependent on a multiplicity of conditions, the results have been greatly divergent among different animal species and even man. For these reasons, it would be illogical and presumptuous to think that one in vitro bioassay model would be able to replace the battery of in vivo systems that now exist. No single model should be expected to be of universal use. Models are different things to different people, and investigators should expect to modify existing models as well as develop new models to add new insight or a new dimension.

In conclusion, the observations that transformation can be quantitated, that it follows a linear relationship with dose, that transformed colonies do produce transformed lines with attributes of neoplastic cells, including the production of tumors, and that in vivo activity correlates with in vitro activity provide evidence that chemically induced carcinogenesis can be studied in vitro.

REFERENCES

1. Hill, J., Cautions against the immoderate use of snuff etc., R. Baldwin, London, 1761; quotations from second edition, London, 1761; and an edition published by J. Potts, Dublin, 1764; rediscovered and published by Redmond, D. E., Jr., Tobacco and cancer: The first clinical report, 1961, *N. Engl. J. Med.,* 282, 18, 1970.
2. Pott, P., Chirurgical observations relative to the cancer of the scrotum, London, 1775; reprinted *Natl. Cancer Inst. Monogr.,* 10, 1963.
3. Yamagiwa, K. and Ichikawa, K., Experimentelle Studie über die Pathogenese der Epithelialgeschwülste, *Mitt. Med. Fak. Tokio,* 15, 295, 1915.
4. Boyland, E., The correlation of experimental carcinogenesis and cancer in men, *Prog. Exp. Tumor Res.,* 11, 222, 1969.
5. Berwald, Y. and Sachs, L., *In vitro* transformation of normal cells to tumor cells by carcinogenic hydrocarbons, *J. Natl. Cancer Inst.,* 35, 641, 1965.
6. DiPaolo, J. A. and Donovan, P. J., Properties of Syrian hamster cells transformed in the presence of carcinogenic hydrocarbons, *Exp. Cell Res.,* 48, 361, 1967.
7. Chen, T. T. and Heidelberger, C., *In vitro* malignant transformation of cells derived from mouse prostate in the presence of 3-methylcholanthrene, *J. Natl. Cancer Inst.,* 42, 915, 1969.
8. DiPaolo, J. A., Takano, K., and Popescu, N. C., Quantitation of chemically induced neoplastic transformation of Balb/3T3 cloned cell lines, *Cancer Res.,* 32, 2686, 1972.
9. DiPaolo, J. A., Donovan, P. J., and Nelson, R., Quantitative studies of *in vitro* transformation by chemical carcinogens, *J. Natl. Cancer Inst.,* 42, 867, 1969.
10. DiPaolo, J. A., Nelson, R. L., and Donovan, P. J., *In vitro* transformation of Syrian hamster embryo cells by diverse chemical carcinogens, *Nature,* 235, 278, 1972.
11. DiPaolo, J. A., Rabson, A. S., and Malmgren, R. A., *In vitro* viral transformation of chemically transformed cells, *J. Natl. Cancer Inst.,* 40, 757, 1968.
11a. Gallo, R. C., Summary of recent observations on the molecular biology of RNA tumor viruses and attempts at application to human leukemia, *Am. J. Clin. Pathol.,* 60, 80, 1973.
12. DiPaolo, J. A., Nelson, R. L., and Donovan, P. J., Sarcoma producing cell lines derived from clones transformed *in vitro* by benzo(a)pyrene, *Science,* 165, 917, 1969.
13. DiPaolo, J. A., Nelson, R. L., and Donovan, P. J., Morphological, oncogenic, and karyological characteristics of Syrian hamster embryo cells transformed *in vitro* by carcinogenic polycyclic hydrocarbons, *Cancer Res.,* 31, 1118, 1971.
14. DiPaolo, J. A., Popescu, N. C., and Nelson, R. L., Chromosomal banding patterns and *in vitro* transformation of Syrian hamster cells, *Cancer Res.,* 33, 3250, 1973.
15. DiPaolo, J. A., Donovan, P. J., and Nelson, R. L., Quantitative studies of *in vitro* transformation by chemical carcinogens, *J. Natl. Cancer Inst.,* 42, 867, 1969.
16. DiPaolo, J. A., Nelson, R. L., Donovan, P. J., and Evans, C. H., Host-mediated *in vivo-in vitro* combination assay system for chemical carcinogenesis, *Arch. Pathol.,* 95, 380, 1973.
17. Casto, B. C., Pieczynski, W. J., and DiPaolo, J. A., Enhancement of adenovirus transformation by pretreatment of hamster cells with carcinogenic polycyclic hydrocarbons, *Cancer Res.,* 33, 919, 1973.
18. DiPaolo, J. A., Donovan, P. J., and Nelson, R. L., X-irradiation enhancement of transformation by benzo[a]pyrene in hamster embryo cells, *Proc. Natl. Acad. Sci. U.S.A.,* 68, 1734, 1973.

CHEMICAL INTERACTION MEASUREMENTS
REPORT OF DISCUSSION GROUP NO. 11

D. S. R. Sarma

BACKGROUND INFORMATION

The overall aim of this report is to discuss and suggest short-term predictive tests for potential chemical carcinogens. It is realized that the method to be adopted should be reliable, economical, and technically simple. No attempts were made to go into the details of the nature of chemical or physical interaction of the chemical carcinogen with the cellular target molecule.

Measurement of induction of tumors, although ideal, is unfortunately time-consuming. Hence, indirect indicator tests for the measurement of chemical interactions in the target molecule were sought. Almost all chemical carcinogens are mutagenic in bacteriophage and bacteria.[1] Hence, induction of mutation in bacteria is often taken as an indirect measure of carcinogenic potential of a chemical.[2,3] Several methods have been described, using microorganisms as test systems to evaluate a chemical for its potential carcinogenic activity.[2-4] However, certain chemicals require mammalian metabolic activation. Hence, the use of animal models becomes important. One of the assays using animal models is the dominant-lethal test.[5] This method consists of the administration of chemicals into the male animal, subsequent mating with an untreated female, and dissection and examination of the pregnant animal. Chromosome aberrations or dominant-lethal mutations cause the death of the embryos. Unfortunately, this method is also time-consuming. Hence, alternate, indirect indicator tests have been and are being developed.

In view of the long latent period between the initial interaction of the chemical carcinogen with cellular molecules and the final biological event, namely the appearance of cancer, it becomes difficult to define the target molecule with which the carcinogen interacts. Further, it also should be realized that such an event alone is not sufficient for the production of cancer. As a working model, the interaction of a chemical with DNA can be studied in the hope that it plays an important role in the initiation of carcinogenesis. It may be possible that an altered protein or RNA may also play key roles in ultimately generating an alteration in DNA structure. The following facts favor the suggestion that DNA is the probable target molecule in the initiation of chemical carcinogenesis:

1. Chemical carcinogens induce mutation in bacteriophage, bacteria, and even in some eukaryotic cells.[2-4]
2. In vivo, there is a long latent period between the initial event, namely the interaction of chemicals with the target molecule, and the final biological event, the appearance of cancer. In eukaryotes, DNA is the primary molecule that can store information for long periods of time, is relatively stable, and has the capacity to self-duplicate.
3. Cells from patients with xeroderma pigmentosum (x-p) exhibit deficiency of UV-induced DNA repair.[6] Such patients are prone to skin cancer when exposed to actinic radiation.
4. Some cocarcinogens inhibit UV-induced DNA repair capacity.[7]
5. Chemical carcinogens do interact with DNA.[8]

A few of the many types of interactions between chemical carcinogens and DNA are listed here.[9,10]

1. Covalent binding of chemical carcinogens with several bases of DNA; e.g., N-7, O-6, and C-8 of deoxyguanosine, N-1 and N-3 of deoxyadenosine, and N-1 of deoxycytosine, etc.
2. Interstrand and intrastrand crosslinks of DNA.
3. Intercalation with DNA bases.
4. Interaction with phosphate and amino groups of DNA.

Many of these interactions, either directly or through the mediation of enzymes, lead to strand breakage, either single- or double-strand breaks.[11-15] Hence, strand breakage may be a useful technique to study the chemical carcinogen interaction with DNA. All four members of the discussion group postulated that virtually all ultimate chemical carcinogens induce DNA damage, which can be measured by proper use of (a) centrifugal techniques, such as sucrose and cesium chloride gradients, and (b) unscheduled DNA synthesis.

USE OF SEDIMENTATION ANALYSIS

Drs. Kanagalingam and Balis, using rat intestine as the experimental model, have shown that methylazoxymethanol acetate and dimethylhydrazine, known intestinal carcinogens, induced DNA breaks, which are distinguishable from the breaks induced by non-carcinogens, as detected on alkaline sucrose gradients. Extensive repair of such damage can be seen within 16 hours after the administration of the carcinogen, which is not the case with non-carcinogens.[16]

Dr. Goodman, employing rat liver as the experimental model, demonstrated that an early effect of ingestion of the hepatic carcinogen 3'-methyl-4-dimethylaminoazobenzene is the occurrence of DNA repair synthesis in hepatic cells. This is evidenced by the production of single-strand breaks in DNA (sucrose gradient centrifugation studies) and non-semiconservative DNA synthesis (cesium chloride gradient centrifugation studies).[17,18]

Drs. Sarma, Cox, Damjanov, Michael, Rajalakshmi, Stewart, Zubroff, and Farber have shown that virtually all chemical carcinogens tested induced single-strand breaks in rat liver DNA in vivo.[11-15] Some hepatocarcinogens, in addition, induced double-strand breaks (Table 1). The time required for repair of single-strand breaks varied, ranging from a few hours to a few weeks. Hepatocarcinogens are at one end of the spectrum, since the damage induced by these agents was not repaired completely even at the end of two weeks. In contrast, the damage induced by chemotherapeutic agents was repaired within four hours. Further, a number of hepatotoxic agents, such as cycloheximide, morpholine, piperidine, piperazine, cyclophosphamide, galactosamine, α-amanitine, isopentenyladenosine, and nitrosocitrulline, did not induce any obvious DNA-strand damage in the liver. Sarma, Rajalakshmi and Farber[10] suggested that a potential hepatocarcinogen either induces double-strand breaks or single-strand breaks that take a long time to be repaired; during this long time, if a cell with damaged DNA replicates, single-strand breaks may become double-strand breaks of greater potential damage.

USE OF UNSCHEDULED DNA SYNTHESIS

Dr. Stich and co-workers, using fibroblasts, have shown that virtually all ultimate carcinogens tested induced unscheduled DNA synthesis (Table

TABLE 1

Effect of Several Chemicals on the Induction of Single-strand Breaks in Hepatic DNA in vivo

Hepatic carcinogens	Non-hepatic carcinogens
Dimethylnitrosamine	N-Methyl-N-nitrosourea
Methylazoxymethanol acetate	N-Methyl-N'-nitro-N-nitrosoguanidine
Diethylnitrosamine	Methylnitrosourethane
2-Acetylaminofluorene	Methylmethanesulfonate
N-Hydroxy-2-acetylaminofluorene*	N-Ethyl-N-nitrosourea
N-Acetoxy-2-acetylaminofluorene*	Ethylmethanesulfonate
N-Nitrosomorpholine*	4-Nitroquinoline N-oxide
N-Nitrosopiperidine	4-Hydroxyaminoquinoline N-oxide
N,N-Dinitrosopiperazine	
3-Hydroxyxanthine*	

	Chemotherapeutic agents
Nitrosodihydrosouracil*	Camptothecin
3'-Methyl-4-dimethylaminoazobenzene	Bleomycin
Aflatoxin B$_1$	Hycanthone methanesulfonate

*These agents, in addition, induced double-strand breaks.

2). They have also documented that the precarcinogens, after being activated by a postmitochondrial liver mixture, could induce unscheduled DNA synthesis. Furthermore, organotropic carcinogens and precarcinogens can be identified by a combined in vivo and in vitro system.[19] The proposed method of applying a compound in vivo and measuring DNA repair synthesis in vitro may detect not only chemicals that require activation by a particular tissue, but may recognize the organs and tissues from which neoplasms arise. All these observations suggest that measurement of DNA damage and repair may be considered as a valid assay for the measurement of chemical carcinogen—DNA interaction.

The two most promising procedures to measure DNA damage and repair appear to be (1) centrifugational analysis, using alkaline and neutral gradients, and (2) the unscheduled incorporation of radioactive precursors into DNA of non-dividing cells with subsequent detection by autoradiography.

ADVANTAGES AND LIMITATIONS OF THE TWO TECHNIQUES

The centrifugation technique has several advantages. Among them are the following: the evidence suggests that this method can be used to distinguish a carcinogen from a non-carcinogen in vivo; it can detect organ-specific carcinogens in vivo; it can determine the damage and repair quantitatively; it takes into account total cellular repair capacity. The main limitation of this method is the

TABLE 2

DNA Repair Synthesis as a Bioassay for Chemical Carcinogens

Unscheduled ^{3}HTdR uptake detected	Unscheduled ^{3}HTdR uptake not detected
4-Nitroquinoline 1-oxide (and 16 carcinogenic derivatives)	7,12-Dimethylbenzanthracene
3-Methyl-4-nitropyridine 1-oxide	Benz[a] pyrene
3-Methyl-4-hydroxyaminopyridine 1-oxide	3-Methylcholanthrene
2,3-Dimethyl-4-nitropyridine-1-oxide	3-Methylcholanthrene 6,7-dihydrodiol
2,3-Dimethyl-4-hydroxyaminopyridine 1-oxide	Dibenz[a,h] anthracene
2-Methyl-4-nitropyridine 1-oxide	Dibenz[a.h] anthracene 3,4-dihydrodiol
3-Ethyl-4-nitropyridine 1-oxide	Benz[a] anthracene
2,3-Diethyl-4-nitropyridine 1-oxide	Benz[a] anthracene 5,6-dihydrodiol
Rugulosin	Dimethylnitrosamine
Patulin	n-Amyl nitrite
N-Methyl-N'-nitro-N-nitrosoguanidine	Cyclophosphamide
Methylmethanesulfonate	Aflatoxin B$_1$
Ethylmethanesulfonate	
Methylnitrosourea	Daunomycin
	Acriflavine, neutral
Nitrogen mustard	Ethidium bromide
1-Butyl hydroperoxide	2-Acetylaminofluorene
	4-Aminostilbene
1CR-191	4-Acetylaminostilbene
	2-Acetylaminophenanthrene
N-Hydroxy-2-acetylaminofluorene	4-Acetylaminobiphenyl
N-Acetoxy-2-acetylaminofluorene	4-Aminobiphenyl
N-Hydroxy-4-acetylaminostilbene	
N-Acetoxy-4-acetylaminostilbene	Cycasin
N-Hydroxy-2-acetylaminophenanthrene	
N-Acetoxy-2-acetylaminophenanthrene	3-Hydroxyxanthine
N-Acetoxy-4-acetylaminobiphenyl	Guanine N-oxide
N-Acetoxy-3-acetylaminofluorene	
N-Myristoyloxy-2-acetylaminofluorene	
Benz[a] anthracene 5,6-epoxide	
3-Methylcholanthrene 6,7-epoxide	

need to pre-label the DNA, which is expensive and sometimes difficult. Currently work is in progress to develop a highly sensitive technique to determine microquantities of DNA.

On the other hand, unscheduled DNA repair synthesis is simple and requires only few cells (approximately 200 cells per sample); it can also be used on cells from human beings (lymphocytes, fibroblasts from skin biopsies, cells from amniocentesis samples); it can be applied to differentiated and non-differentiated cells; it permits the visualization of DNA repair in individual nuclei; it can reveal variations within a cell population; it is highly economical and can be completed within a ten-day period (or within two days if the rapid autoradiographic method is employed). This method, however, has certain limitations: it does not assay for polynucleotide ligase activity; it does not identify to what extent the damage is repaired; it does not distinguish between single- and double-strand breaks; it measures only excision repair, which is one of the many repair processes that the cell may be adopting; and it cannot be applied to rapidly proliferating tissues.

These methods may pull some non-carcinogens into the carcinogen group. Any agent that induces DNA damage must be viewed with great suspicion. It is possible that a chemical interaction that does not lead to DNA-strand breakage will not be detected.

A Proposed Method of Using DNA Damage and Repair as a Bioassay, Using Sucrose Gradients

The liver DNA of white male rats of the Wistar strain (Carworth Farms), weighing approximately 100 g, is pre-labeled by injecting tritiated thymidine (^{3}HTdR), sp. act. 20 Ci/mmole, intraperitoneally at a dose of 50 μCi every 4 hours, beginning 18 hours after partial hepatectomy, for a total of 450 μCi. The animals are allowed to recover for at least two weeks before being given the compound under study.[11] In cases where intestine is used as the experimental model, intestinal DNA can be labeled by administering ^{3}HTdR 24 hours prior to using the animal.[16] Alternatively, to label the DNA of several organs, ^{3}HTdR is administered to baby rats from day 1 to day 20 after birth; two to three days after the last injection of ^{3}HTdR the animals can be used.

Each compound has to be tested for optimal dose and time, carefully avoiding any dose that induces cell necrosis over the time-span studied.

Water-insoluble compounds can be given in dimethylsulfoxide; care should be taken, however, not to administer more than 1 to 2 ml of dimethylsulfoxide.

A whole-cell suspension of liver in EDTA (ethylenediaminetetraacetic acid) is rapidly prepared mechanically by the use of a spatula. About 2 g of liver is used in a petri dish with 1 ml of cold 0.024M EDTA and 0.075M NaCl buffer, pH 7.5. The preparation, consisting of clumps and individual liver cells, is centrifuged for 1 minute at 200 rpm at 4°. The supernatant contains a suspension of liver cells. The number of cells is counted in a hemocytometer, and the amount of DNA is measured by the diphenylamine method of Burton.

Alkaline or neutral sucrose gradients are prepared in cellulose nitrate tubes (diameter 9/16″ and length 3 3/4″). Quantities of 5 ml linear alkaline sucrose gradients (5 to 20%) containing 0.9M NaCl are prepared over a 1-ml shelf of 2.3M sucrose. A lysing solution (0.3 ml) of 0.30M NaCl, 0.03M EDTA, 0.1M Tris-HCl buffer and 0.5% sodium dodecyl sulfate, pH 12.5, is carefully layered on top of the gradient. The lysing agent for neutral sucrose gradients is the same as that used for alkaline gradients, except that the pH is 7.5. A volume of cells ranging from 0.01 to 0.3 ml and consisting of approximately 1 μg of DNA (about 300 to 500 cpm) is added to the tube. Another aliquot (0.1 ml) of lysing agent is added on the top of the cells to insure complete lysis, and the rest of the tube is filled with mineral oil. Five to ten minutes later the gradients are centrifuged at 25,000 rpm for 30 minutes at 20°, using the Beckman SW 40 rotor in a Spinco model L2-65B ultracentrifuge. The rotor is decelerated to a stop without the brake. Fractions of 20 drops are collected from the bottom of each pierced tube by pumping mineral oil from the top. The first two fractions comprise the 2.3M sucrose shelf. Bovine serum albumin (20 μg) is added to each fraction before precipitating it with 4 ml of cold 5% TCA. Acid-precipitable radioactivity in each fraction is determined. It may be noted that the size of gradient and the type of centrifuge tube can be altered.

This method can be applied to other organs as well, such as kidney, lung, brain, and intestine. Because of the presence of different types of nucleases in intestines, one has to be careful. As pointed out by Drs. Kanagalingam and Balis, this difficulty can be overcome by anesthetizing the rat to dull the intestines prior to removal and by increasing the speed of operation.[16]

A Proposed Schedule of Using DNA Repair Synthesis as a Bioassay

Step 1

Add different concentrations of the test chemical to monolayer cultures of non-dividing mammalian cells for 1 to 3 hours and estimate the unscheduled incorporation of ^{3}HTdR (10 μCi/ml for 90 minutes).[20] If no DNA repair synthesis can be detected, proceed with Step 2.

Step 2

Mix the test chemical with an activation preparation (fortified postmitochondrial liver fraction).[19] Add this mixture to monolayer cultures of non-dividing mammalian cells and estimate the unscheduled incorporation of ^{3}HTdR. If no DNA repair synthesis can be detected, proceed with Step 3.

Step 3

Add the test chemical to tiny pieces of various mammalian organs for 1 to 5 hours, then place these organ pieces for 90 minutes into ^{3}HTdR-containing culture medium.[21] If no DNA repair can be detected, proceed with Step 4.

Step 4

Apply the combined in vivo/in vitro system. Six-week-old male mice are injected with varying doses of the test chemical. Two hours after the injection various organs are removed, teased into tiny pieces, then incubated in standard tissue culture medium containing 10 μCi/ml tritiated thymidine (20 Ci/mmole) for 3 hours at 37°C, fixed with a mixture of alcohol and acetic acid (3:1), squashed between cover slips and microscopic slides, stained with 0.2% acetoorcein solution, coated with Kodak NTB-3 emulsion, and exposed for two weeks. The incorporation of ^{3}HTdR into nuclear DNA has to be checked by treating squash preparations with deoxyribonuclease prior to autoradiography. The incorporation of ^{3}HTdR into DNA will be taken as a measure of repair synthesis.

CONCLUSION

The data described in this report suggest that use of DNA damage and repair is an economical, rapid, and relevant indicator for chemical carcinogens and precarcinogens. The idea is based on the assumption that chemical carcinogens interact with DNA and that the ensuing DNA damage will result in DNA repair. The methods described have the potential to differentiate carcinogens from non-carcinogens; they can detect organ-specific carcinogens in vivo; they can be used on mammalian cells, including human ones; they can be quantitative; and they can be completed in a relatively short time period. These procedures, as they exist now, may not replace the standard direct tests for carcinogenicity, but they may be useful as a rapid prescreening tool.

REFERENCES

1. Miller, E. C. and Miller, J. A., in *Chemical Mutagens,* Vol. 1, Hollaender, A., Ed., Plenum Press, New York, 1971, 83.
2. Ames, B. N., Lee, F. D., and Durston, W. E., *Proc. Natl. Acad. Sci.,* 70, 782, 1973.
3. Ames, B. N., Durston, W. E., Yamasaki, E., and Lee, F. D., *Proc. Natl. Acad. Sci.,* 70, 2281, 1973.
4. Legator, M. S. and Malling, H. V., in *Chemical Mutagens,* Vol. 2, Hollaender, A., Ed., Plenum Press, New York, 1971, 569.
5. Bateman, A. J. and Epstein, S. S., in *Chemical Mutagens,* Vol. 2, Hollaender, A., Ed., Plenum Press, New York, 1971, 541.
6. Cleaver, J. E., *Proc. Natl. Acad. Sci.,* 63, 428, 1969.
7. Gaudin, D., Gregg, R. S., and Yielding, K. I., *Biochem. Biophys. Res. Commun.,* 45, 630, 1971.
8. Miller, J. A., *Cancer Res.,* 30, 559, 1970.
9. Irving, C. C., in *Methods in Cancer Research,* Vol. 7, Busch, H., Ed., Academic Press, New York, 1973, 189.
10. Sarma, D. S. R., Rajalakshmi, S., and Farber, E., in *Cancer. A Comprehensive Treatise,* Vol. 1, Becker, F. F., Ed., Plenum Press, New York, in press.
11. Cox, R., Damjanov, I., Abanobi, S. E., and Sarma, D. S. R., *Cancer Res.,* 33, 2114, 1973.
12. Damjanov, I., Cox, R., Sarma, D. S. R., and Farber, E., *Cancer Res.,* 33, 2122, 1973.
13. Stewart, B. W., Farber, E., and Mirvish, S. S. *Biochem. Biophys. Res. Commun.,* 53, 773, 1973.
14. Stewart, B. W. and Farber, E., *Cancer Res.,* 33, 3209, 1973.
15. Rajalakshmi, S. and Sarma, D. S. R., *Biochem. Biophys. Res. Commun.,* 53, 1268, 1973.
16. Kanagalingam, K. and Balis, M. E., *Proc. Am. Assoc. Cancer Res.,* 15, 46, 1974.
17. Goodman, J. I. and Potter, V. R., *Cancer Res.,* 32, 766, 1972.
18. Goodman, J. I., *Biochem. Biophys. Res. Commun.,* 56, 52, 1974.
19. Laishes, B. and Stich, H. F., *Biochem. Biophys. Res. Commun.,* 52, 827, 1973.
20. Lieberman, M. W., Baney, R. N., Lee, R. E., Sell, S., and Farber, E., *Cancer Res.,* 31, 1297, 1971.
21. Lieberman, M. W. and Forbes, P. D., *Nat. New Biol.,* 241, 199, 1973.

SECTION 17
REPORT OF DISCUSSION GROUP NO. 12
MUTAGENESIS ASSESSMENT

Frederick J. de Serres

I. INTRODUCTION

An acceptable prescreen test procedure must possess certain specific characteristics to be minimally acceptable. The test must be rapid, it must be relatively inexpensive, and it must be reasonably easy to perform. It must also be validated; that is to say, the results obtained must be shown to be reproducible in different laboratories. A useful prescreen for carcinogenesis must not generate false negatives and must limit greatly the number of false positives that arise. It is necessary, as will be pointed out later, to use a battery of tests, but the number of tests employed should be limited so as not to contribute excessively to an unacceptably large number of false positives.

The National Cancer Institute has begun an effort in which it will seek to prescreen some 85 compounds (including representative procarcinogens, activated carcinogens, non-carcinogens and non-carcinogenic mutagens) in three different assay systems that are capable of measuring genetic effects. The three systems are the microbial host-mediated assay, mammalian cells in tissue culture using specific-locus mutational assay systems, and excision repair of DNA damage in mammalian cells. In all instances efforts will be made to provide for mammalian metabolic activation. This study will seek to ascertain the extent to which the above-specified mutational assay systems might serve to effectively prescreen carcinogens.

It is recognized that, while the information forthcoming from the NCI effort will provide additional perspective, such studies are not sufficient in scope to provide a final assessment of the relationship of carcinogenicity to mutagenicity. Attention is further called to the fact that certain of the systems proposed as a possible prescreen are not as yet fully understood with respect to their mechanism of action.

A wide variety of assay systems, including several new procedures, are under active development pursuant to the goal of providing an assessment of the mutagenic potential of chemicals.

Many types of genetic damage can be produced by genetically active substances, but there is no single test that can detect all possible genetic effects. Each of the proposed assay systems suffers from the defect that it fails to provide a complete evaluation of all possible genetic events. Thus, for these purposes a battery of tests is generally recommended that would include both mammalian and sub-mammalian assay systems.

Mutagenicity tests of chemical carcinogens have shown that many carcinogens are genetically active. The correlation is by no means complete, nor are short-term tests for mutagenicity sufficiently tested to indicate whether they can be utilized to predict accurately carcinogenic activity in man. While there are provocative results showing great promise, much additional work is needed, such as the NCI effort.

This paper attempts to review the following: assay systems developed to detect various types of genetic activity; the results of tests with known chemical carcinogens; and the potential value of the most promising systems as a predictive test for carcinogenic activity in man.

For each of the assay systems, the utility of the assay can be enhanced by a simple modification of the testing protocol that makes it possible not only to test the initial substance but also its metabolites. Many of the sub-mammalian assay systems cannot perform the same metabolic conversions that take place in mammalian systems, but by placing indicator organisms in the peritoneum of a mammal, as in the host-mediated assay, or by utilizing various in vitro activation systems (that utilize microsomes from mammalian or human liver), the sensitivity of the assay can be markedly enhanced.

Apparently, many carcinogens are mutagens, but not all mutagens are demonstrable carcinogens. To gain an understanding of this apparent anomaly, and to narrow down our battery of tests to a single test system or at least to a few test systems that can predict carcinogenic activity in man, data have to be collected in a way that enables us to determine whether carcinogens produce a particular type of genetic alteration. If, for example, carcinogens only produce a particular type of genetic alteration, our assays could be restricted to the detection of this particular class alteration. By making the assays for mutagenic activity in a wide range of organisms, from bacterial cells to human cells in culture, the simplest assays that would provide the desired information could then be used with confidence in routine screening programs.

II. SUB-MAMMALIAN ASSAY SYSTEMS TO DETECT MUTAGENIC ACTIVITY

A. Repair-deficient Strains of Bacteria

At present the usefulness of the rapid-screening tests first described by Rosenkranz and his associates,[2,3] which use DNA polymerase-deficient mutants of *Escherichia coli*, appears to be largely limited to the detection of direct-acting alkylating agents. No positive results have yet been obtained with procarcinogenic aromatic amines, polycyclic hydrocarbons, and AAF or its derivatives. Attempts to activate these compounds with rat liver extracts supplemented with cofactors were unsuccessful. Further, a false positive result was obtained with caffeine.

Conclusions and Recommendations

Since the test appears to depend on such factors as diffusion of the test compound on the agar plate, absence of interaction with media constituents, and chemical stability, it is recommended that modifications of this test be investigated with the aim of overcoming these limitations. Some of the modifications proposed were (1) tests for growth in liquid culture, (2) use of minimal-nutrient media sufficient to support adequate growth, (3) separation of the activation step from the test step, and (4) use of additional indicator organisms. It was agreed that in its present form the test fails to suffice as a prescreen for carcinogenicity.

B. *Salmonella*

A tester set of histidine-requiring mutants has been developed by Ames and co-workers[3-5] to determine whether particular types of genetic alterations can be produced by a particular agent. Three of the strains in the tester set (TA 1531, TA 1532, and TA 1534) are designed to detect various types of frameshift mutations. A fourth strain (TA

1530) detects mutagens that cause base-pair substitutions. The mutations in the three frameshift testers all occur at so-called "hot spots" in the histidine locus, and their high rates of reversion make them especially sensitive indicators of this type of genetic activity. All four strains also have a defective excision-repair system, which makes them additionally sensitive to any mutagen that alters DNA in a way that would normally be repaired by this system.[3] The tests are usually performed by adding a few crystals or an aqueous solution of the chemical under study as a spot to a uniform lawn of one of the histidine-requiring mutants on the surface of a petri plate containing minimal medium.

In early tests[4] with seven epoxides of carcinogenic polycyclic hydrocarbons, strain TA 1532 reverted after treatment with two of the carcinogens, but not the other five. A so-called deep rough derivative of TA 1532 was then constructed, which removes most of the lipopolysaccharide coat. The sensitivity of the new strain (TA 1537) was enhanced, as evidenced by the observation that three of the original seven epoxides now showed genetic activity. In subsequent papers, deep rough derivatives of all four of the original strains were deployed to test the mutagenicity of certain polycyclic aromatic compounds.[3,5] Most of these were shown to react with testers TA 1537 or TA 1538, indicating that they cause frameshift mutations. These studies and later work involving liver homogenates to achieve in vitro metabolic activation have shown that many carcinogens and/or their metabolites prove to be mutagenic.

To determine whether potent carcinogens are potent mutagens, we need to know the effect of treatment with a carcinogen on a forward-mutation system and to determine the increase in mutation rate over that occurring spontaneously. Obviously, such a comparison would be meaningless with the *Salmonella* system, because it is a reverse-mutational assay rather than a forward-mutational assay, and because the genetic activity is markedly enhanced by selecting mutants that occur at "hot spots" and by making all strains deficient for excision repair. Indeed, Ames[4] has shown that chemicals that are "potent" mutagens in his reverse-mutational assay are either only weakly mutagenic or not mutagenic at all upon performing forward-mutational assays (resistance to a proline analog). In addition, there is evidence that certain mutagenic compounds, such as ICR-

170, are only weakly mutagenic in the *Salmonella* reversion assay while they have proven to be potent mutagens both in *Drosophila* and in *Neurospora* when forward-mutational analysis is used. There is also evidence that certain mutagens claimed to cause only frameshift mutations in *Salmonella* produce predominantly base-pair substitutions in *Neurospora*.

Conclusions and Recommendations

The Salmonella tester set is a highly promising system for rapid, simple, and inexpensive detection of genetic activity. Lack of concurrence with assay systems in eukaryotic organisms may be resolved by selecting additional histidine-requiring mutants as testers, particularly those capable of detecting base-pair substitutions. There is concern that the utilization of this assay system may result in the erroneous classification of chemicals with regard to their quantitative and qualitative effects, since the test only measures reverse mutation of a highly selected set of testers biased in favor of frameshift mutations rather than forward mutations. The practical utility contended by this assay awaits completion of the NCI investigation described above, wherein carcinogens and their inactive homologs will be tested for mutagenicity. No further recommendation for deployment of this system is possible until the results of the above study are known.

C. Yeast

In the diploid yeast *Saccharomyces cerevisiae,* strains heterozygous for a series of linked genetic markers can be used to determine the frequency of mitotic recombination. If the markers are non-allelic, intergenic recombination can be studied; if allelic markers are used, intragenic recombination (or gene conversion) can be studied. Various diploid strains have been developed. In the newest strain, D5, two different complementing hetero-alleles at the *ad-2* locus are used. One allele is leaky and forms pink colonies as a homozygous diploid; the other is non-leaky and forms red colonies. Normal diploid colonies are white; when intergenic recombination has taken place, pink- and red-sectored colonies are found.

Assays for mitotic recombination have been made by Zimmerman,[27] and a high percentage of selected substances tested has been found to induce mitotic recombination. The molecular basis for the mechanism responsible for this activity is not well understood, but the simplicity of the assay system would make it an especially useful screen for mutagenic activity.

Conclusions

The system is known to respond to a wide range of mutagenic substances and provides useful quantitative information regarding genetic damage.

Recommendation

The assay system should be used with appropriate metabolic activation to evaluate a large number of known carcinogens for the purpose of determining the extent of positive correlation between mitotic recombination and carcinogenic activity.

D. Neurospora

A two-component heterokaryon of *Neurospora crassa* has been developed,[26] which is heterozygous for two closely linked loci in the *ad-3* region. Mutants at the *ad-3A* and *ad-3B* locus have a requirement for adenine and can be selected directly on the basis of their accumulation of a reddish-purple pigment in the mycelium. The *ad-3* mutations can be characterized by a series of simple genetic tests to distinguish point mutations from deletions and to obtain a presumptive identification of the genetic alterations in the point mutations at the *ad-3B* locus at the molecular level.

Studies with a group of ten carcinogens,[20a] including diepoxides, naphthylamines, aflatoxins, and ethyleneimine, have shown positive correlation between carcinogenic and mutagenic activity. Genetic characterization of the point mutations at the *ad-3B* locus indicates that chemical carcinogens produce gene mutations as a result of a wide variety of genetic alterations, the most frequent alteration being point mutations resulting from base-pair substitution.[20b]

Conclusions

The above system shows real promise for the evaluation of the mutagenicity of chemical carcinogens. The level of effort required for this undertaking is akin to that of most mammalian-cell systems. Since the assay is based on analysis of forward mutation, it should eventually be possible to determine the quantitative nature of the correlation between carcinogenic and mutagenic activity (e.g., are potent carcinogens potent mutagens in *Neurospora*?). In addition, the capability of characterizing the mutants genetically will make it possible to determine whether carcinogens produce particular types of genetic alterations. This type of information is essential for the effective interpretation of mutagenic data as it relates to cancer risk.

Recommendations

Larger numbers of chemical carcinogens and non-carcinogenic chemicals should be tested with appropriate metabolic activation pursuant to an evaluation of the method's utility as a prescreen procedure.

III. ASSAYS TO DETECT GENE MUTATIONS IN CULTURED MAMMALIAN CELLS

Since the demonstration in 1968 of mutational activity in mammalian cells grown in tissue culture,[9,16] it was quickly recognized that the cell-culture system would be ideally suited for testing the mutagenicity of chemical compounds in man's environment. It was also considered that a direct assay of mammalian or human somatic cells would provide a better estimation of possible genetic hazards of chemicals in man. Furthermore, there is the added advantage that the same cells used for the induction of mutations can also be employed for neoplastic transformation. Cultured mammalian cells thus offer an opportunity to test the possible relationship between the processes of mutagenesis and carcinogenesis.

The types of somatic cells that have been employed for mutation studies include both human and non-human mammalian cells of either normal or tumor origin. For the present purpose, studies with Chinese hamster cells, mouse lymphoma cells, and diploid tumor cells will be briefly summarized. As detailed below, each cell type possesses certain advantages and limitations, either from a theoretical or from a technical point of view. While initial efforts with cultured mammalian cells in mutational assays appear to be highly encouraging, further technical developments are necessary to make these tests more reliable and meaningful.

A. Chinese Hamster Cells

Cell lines derived from the lung, ovary, and other tissues of Chinese hamster (*Cricetulus griseus,* 2n = 22) usually maintain a near-diploid chromosome number and exhibit active growth and high cloning efficiency. Selective media have been developed to detect both forward and reverse mutations at three genetic loci involving enzymes in the salvage pathways of purines and pyrimidines. In Chinese hamster, as in man, the utilization of preformed hypoxanthine and guanine is controlled by an X-linked gene. Mutant cells at this locus are deficient in the enzyme hypoxanthine-guanine phosphoribosyl transferase (HGPRT) and are resistant to certain purine analogues. Similarly, mutant cells deficient in adenine phosphoribosyl transferase (APRT) cannot metabolize preformed adenine or its analogues for incorporation into nucleic acids. The third type of drug-resistant mutants commonly studied in these and other mammalian cells are those deficient in thymidine kinase (TK). Such cells exhibit resistance to the thymidine analogue 5-bromodeoxyuridine. Both APRT and TK activities appear to be controlled by autosomal genes in man, and it is likely that this is true of other mammals as well.

Cells carrying mutations at these loci can be selected from the wild-type population subjected to an environment containing an appropriate purine or pyrimidine analogue. Revertants to the wild type can be recovered in selective media, in which the cells are supplied with the natural purines or pyrimidines while the normal *de novo* pathway of purine or pyrimidine biosynthesis is inhibited with an antimetabolite.

It has been demonstrated that Chinese hamster cells, upon treatment with physical (X-rays, ultraviolet light) or chemical (alkylating agents) mutagens, undergo a significant increase in the frequency of forward and reverse mutations over the spontaneous frequency.[6,7] Tests with several representative chemical carcinogens (polycyclic hydrocarbons, aromatic amines, nitroso compounds, and epoxides) and their structurally related non-carcinogenic analogues indicated a positive association between the carcinogenicity and mutagenicity of chemical substances.[8,12–15,19]

B. Mouse Lymphoma Cells

Mouse lymphoma L5178Y cells have been extensively used for oncological, virological, pharmacological, molecular, and toxicological studies over a number of years. There is a massive amount of information available concerning single-cell cloning and in-depth quantitative analysis of these tumor cells. The karyotype of this cell line is essentially diploid. Spontaneous variation with respect to drug sensitivity and nutritional requirement have been observed within its cell populations. Recent experiments indicate the feasibility of experimentally inducing what appear to be gene mutations in these cells. Forward mutations from TK +/- cells to TK -/- have been induced after treatment of cells with X-rays or chemical mutagens.[10] This marker system has also been used to demonstrate the mutagenicity of the drug hycanthone.

Although the cells are tumorous, there is no reason to believe that the mutagenic mechanics in tumor cells should be fundamentally different from those in normal cells. In fact, the induced-mutation rate at the TK locus, as noted above, was found to be similar to the rates found in other mammalian cells in culture or in mouse spermatogonia. Furthermore, the fact that these cells can be grown either in vivo or in vitro makes them particularly suitable for host-mediated mutagenicity tests.

C. Diploid Human Cells

Forward mutations to HGPRT deficiency (resistance to 8-azaguanine) in normal diploid human fibroblasts in culture have been shown to occur either spontaneously[11] or after X-irradiation.[1,2] Some of the mutant isolates have been characterized with respect to their growth response in appropriate media as well as to the properties of phosphoribosyl transferase. These mutant cells resemble closely the cultured fibroblasts derived from patients with Lesch-Nyhan syndrome. This observation strongly supports the contention that such presumptive mutants are indeed true mutations, occurring at the X-linked locus.

Mutations at other loci can, of course, be sought in human diploid cells, providing that selective procedures for specific changes in cellular phenotype are available. Experiments are now under way in Robert DeMars' laboratory at the University of Wisconsin to isolate forward mutations at the adenine phosphoribosyl transferase (APRT) locus, making use of fibroblasts derived from heterozygous carriers whose genotypes had been previously determined.

More recently, chemical induction of forward mutation from HGPRT$^+$ to HGPRT$^-$ in human

lymphoblastoid cell lines has been reported.[22] These long-term lymphocyte lines are derived from normal individuals and are potentially very useful for genetic experiments because of their indefinite life span and the stability of their karyotype, albeit aberrant.

Conclusions and Recommendations

The demonstration of induction of gene mutations in cultured human and non-human mammalian cells has opened many new avenues of research in somatic-cell genetics. At present, it is possible to use several available selective systems for testing the mutagenicity of suspect mutagens. It is obvious that normal human diploid cells are most desirable for these tests, but current studies suggest that reliable conclusions can be drawn from results with non-human mammalian cells.

Additional technical improvements are required if the human-cell system is to be readily amenable to genetic experiments involving induction rates. It appears that the long-term lymphoblastoid cell lines have the greatest potential for these purposes. Due to the demonstrated variation in mutability from locus to locus in experimental organisms, additional selective procedures at different loci should be developed in human and other mammalian cells. It is imperative to ascertain that phenotypic variations observed in cells in vitro are due to genetic rather than epigenetic effects. Where selective methods are available for forward and reverse mutations, attempts should be made to define, by reversion tests with specific mutagens, the nature of molecular alterations at the mutational site. Finally, further developments should be encouraged to utilize a greater number of specific mutagens and to establish the nature of molecular alterations at the mutational site. It is obvious that mammalian metabolism must be provided for, and the inclusion of mammalian cells as indicator organisms in host-mediated mutagenicity assays is to be strongly encouraged.

IV. ASSAYS TO DETECT DNA REPAIR IN CULTURED MAMMALIAN CELLS

Several laboratories have reported an increased repair of cellular DNA following exposure to chemical carcinogens either in vivo or in vitro. This increased repair has been measured either by ^{14}C-labeled-thymidine uptake into DNA or by the linkage of broken DNA strands. A large number of compounds have been tested in vitro regarding their ability to stimulate thymidine uptake into non-replicating DNA.

The cell lines tested have included mouse fibroblasts and human lymphocytes. With a series of 4-nitroquinoline-N-oxide derivatives an excellent correlation has been observed between carcinogenic activity and the ability to stimulate thymidine uptake. With aromatic amines, however, only the "activated" carcinogens stimulated the thymidine uptake in vitro. Thus the test must still be linked to appropriate metabolic activating systems. Initial attempts to do this have demonstrated that administration of carcinogenic nitrosamines to rats led to an increase of thymidine uptake into the non-replicating DNA of target tissues of animals treated with acute doses of carcinogens, rather than into the DNA of insensitive tissues.

Conclusions and Recommendations

In vitro stimulation of thymidine uptake into non-replicating DNA appears to be ready for evaluation as a potential prescreen for chemical carcinogens. The major block to be overcome is that of in vitro metabolic activation.

The in vivo repair measured by either chain linkage or thymidine uptake offers a promising approach to carcinogen prescreening. However, until further data are published on each of these techniques, it is premature to recommend their use as a prescreen.

REFERENCES

1. **Albertini, R. J. and DeMars, R.,** Diploid azaguanine-resistant mutants of cultured human fibroblasts, *Science,* 169, 482, 197.
2. **Albertini, R. J. and DeMars, R.,** Somatic cell mutation. Detection and quantification of X-ray-induced mutation in cultured, diploid human fibroblasts, *Mutat. Res.,* 18, 199, 1973.
3. **Ames, B. N., Gurney, E. G., Miller, J. A., and Bartsch, H.,** Carcinogens as frameshift mutagens: Metabolites and derivatives of 2-acetylaminofluorene and other aromatic amine carcinogens, *Proc. Natl. Acad. Sci. U.S.A.,* 69, 3128, 1972.
4. **Ames, B. N., Lee, F. D., and Durston, W. E.,** An improved bacterial test system for the detection and classification of mutagens and carcinogens, *Proc. Natl. Acad. Sci. U.S.A.,* 70, 782, 1973.
5. **Ames, B. N., Durston, W. E., Yamasaki, E., and Lee, F. D.,** Carcinogens are mutagens: A simple test system combining liver homogenates for activation and bacteria for detection, *Proc. Natl. Acad. Sci. U.S.A.,* 70, 2281, 1973.
6. **Bridges, B. A. and Huckle, J.,** Mutagenesis of cultured mammalian cells by X-radiation and ultraviolet light, *Mutat. Res.,* 10, 141, 1970.
7. **Chu, E. H. Y.,** Mammalian cell genetics. III. Characterization of X-ray-induced forward mutations in Chinese hamster cell cultures, *Mutat. Res.,* 11, 23, 1971.
8. **Chu, E. H. Y.,** Mutagenesis in mammalian cells, in *Environment and Cancer,* Williams and Wilkins, Baltimore, 1972, 198.
9. **Chu, E. H. Y. and Malling, H. V.,** Mammalian cell genetics. II. Chemical induction of specific locus mutations in Chinese hamster cells *in vitro, Proc. Natl. Acad. Sci. U.S.A.,* 61, 1306, 1968.
10. **Clive, D., Flamm, W. G., and Machesko, M. R.,** Mutagenicity of hycanthone in mammalian cells, *Mutat. Res.,* 14, 262, 1972.
11. **DeMars, R. and Held, K. R.,** The spontaneous azaguanine-resistant mutants of diploid human fibroblasts, *Humangenetik,* 16, 87, 1972.

12. Duncan, M. E. and Brookes, P., The induction of azaguanine-resistant mutants in cultured Chinese hamster cells by reactive derivatives of carcinogenic hydrocarbons, *Mutat. Res.,* 21, 107, 1973.

13. Huberman, E., Aspiras, L., Heidelberger, C., Grover, P. L., and Sims, P., Mutagenicity to mammalian cells of epoxides and other derivatives of polycyclic hydrocarbons, *Proc. Natl. Acad. Sci. U.S.A.,* 68, 3195, 1971.

14. Huberman, E., Donovan, P. J., and DiPaolo, J. A., Mutation and transformation of cultured mammalian cells by N-acetoxy-N-2-fluorenylacetamide, *J. Natl. Cancer Inst.,* 48, 837, 1972.

15. Kao, F.-T. and Puck, T. T., Genetics of somatic mammalian cells. VII. Induction and isolation of nutritional mutants in Chinese hamster cells, *Proc. Natl. Acad. Sci. U.S.A.,* 60, 1275, 1968.

16. Kao, F.-T. and Puck, T. T., Genetics of somatic mammalian cells. IX. Quantitation of mutagenesis by physical and chemical agents, *J. Cell. Physiol.,* 74, 245, 1969.

17. Kao, F.-T. and Puck, T. T., Genetics of somatic mammalian cells. XII. Mutagenesis by carcinogenic nitroso compounds, *J. Cell. Physiol.,* 78, 139, 1971.

18. Lieberman, M. W., Baney, R. N., Lee, R. E., Sell, S., and Farber, E., Studies on DNA repair in human lymphocytes treated with proximate carcinogens and alkylating agents, *Cancer Res.,* 31, 1297, 1971.

19. Malling, H. V. and Chu, E. H. Y., Development of mutational model systems for study of carcinogenesis, in *Proceedings of World Symposium on Model Studies in Chemical Carcinogenesis,* October 31 to November 3, 1972, Baltimore, in press.

20. Michael, R. O. and Sarma, D. S. R., Measurement ot *in vivo* damage and repair of rat liver DNA induced by chemical carcinogens, *Proc. Am. Assoc. Cancer Res.,* 14, 5, 1973.

20a. Ong, T.-M. and de Serres, F. J., Mutagenicity of chemical carcinogens in *Neurospora crassa, Cancer Res.,* 32, 1890, 1973.

20b. Ong, T.-M. and de Serres, F. J., Genetic characterization of *ad-3* mutants induced by chemical carcinogens, 1-phenyl-3-monomethyltriazene and 1-phenyl-3,3-dimethyltriazene in *Neurospora crassa, Mutat. Res.,* 20, 17, 1973.

21. Ruelius, H. W., Poirier, L. A., and Fluck, E., unpublished observations.

22. Sato, K., Slesinski, R. S., and Littlefield, J. W., Chemical mutagenesis at the phosphoribosyltransferase locus in cultured human lymphoblasts, *Proc. Natl. Acad. Sci. U.S.A.,* 69, 1244, 1972.

23. Slater, E. E., Anderson, M. D., and Rosenkranz, H. S., Rapid detection of mutagens and carcinogens, *Cancer Res.,* 31, 970, 1971.

24. Stich, H. F., Kieser, D., Laishes, B. A., and San, R. H. C., The use of DNA repair in the identification of carcinogens, precarcinogens and target tissue, *Proc. Can. Cancer Res. Conf.,* in press, 1973.

25. Stich, H. F. and Laishes, B. A., DNA repair and chemical carcinogens, in *Pathobiology Annual,* Vol. 3, Ioachim, H. L., Ed., Appleton Crofts, New York, 1973, 341.

26. Webber, B. B. and de Serres, F. J., Induction kinetics and genetic analysis of X-ray induced mutations in the *ad-3* region of *Neurospora crassa, Proc. Natl. Acad. Sci. U.S.A.,* 53, 430, 1965.

27. Zimmermann, F. K., Induction of mitotic gene conversion by mutagens, *Mutat. Res.,* 11, 327, 1971.

SECTION 18
REPORT OF DISCUSSION GROUP NO. 13
TISSUE CULTURE TECHNIQUES

Bernard Weinstein

Perhaps the most promising new systems for the bioassay of chemical carcinogens, and for analysis of their mechanisms of action, are mammalian cell cultures in which the cells become tumorigenic following exposure to chemical carcinogens. The major systems currently available are (1) hamster embryo primary or secondary cultures;[1,5-7] (2) mouse fibroblast cell lines;[2,3,11] (3) epithelial cells derived from adult rat liver.[10,12,13,16,17]

All of these systems employ rodent cell cultures; there are no published reports on transformation of primate cell cultures with chemical carcinogens.

In the cell-culture assays, it is important to distinguish *morphologic transformation* from *malignant transformation.* The latter term should be reserved to describe cells that are proven to be tumorigenic when injected into appropriate host animals.

Each of the available cell-culture systems has advantages and disadvantages as bioassay for potential carcinogens. The hamster embryo system, originally described by Berwald and Sachs[1] and extensively studied by Dr. DiPaolo's laboratory,[5-7] has the following advantages: (1) the cells are mainly diploid; (2) they have been in culture a minimum number of generations, and therefore may be closer to normal than long-established cell lines; (3) the transformation can be scored quantitatively on individual colonies and within eight days. A disadvantage is that the initial cell population is heterogeneous in cell type and is derived from different embryos. The system also requires considerable experience for precise scoring. Freeman, Huebner and their colleagues[8,9] have described the transformation of rat embryo cultures by various chemical carcinogens, both in the absence and in the presence of murine leukemia viruses. This system has not been scored in a highly quantitative manner, but it may provide the basis for developing a quantitative bioassay for chemical carcinogens, especially since they interact in cells with viruses.

Three mouse fibroblast cell lines are now available for assaying malignant transformation: mouse prostate fibroblasts, BALB/c3T3 cells, and a cell line designated 10T½ derived from C3H mouse embryos. The fibroblast cell lines have the following advantages: (1) they are cloned, thus providing a homogeneous cell population; (2) morphologic transformation is easily and quantitatively scored; (3) the cells are derived from highly inbred strains of mice, thereby permitting precise control of immunogenic, genetic, and viral factors that may influence carcinogen susceptibility. On the other hand, these cell lines have been selected for prolonged growth in culture, are aneuploid, and therefore cannot be considered completely normal. Nevertheless, unless exposed to carcinogens, they are not tumorigenic. Transformation can be scored within one week after exposure to carcinogens in the 3T3 system, and within three to six weeks in the 10T½ cell system.

Approximately 80% of human tumors arise from epithelial cells. It is important, therefore, to develop epithelial cultures from specific tissues, which can be used for quantitative studies on carcinogenesis in cell culture. Several laboratories have now established cell lines from normal adult rat liver that have the hallmarks of epithelial cells. The criteria used to score for transformation of the previously described embryo or fibroblast cultures are not entirely applicable to these epithelial cells.

Early changes noted in the transformation of epithelial cells include loss of adhesiveness, irregularity of the contour of the colony edge, pleomorphism, and increased growth rate and saturation density. Growth in soft agar has been found to be a simple and objective criterion for detecting transformation of epithelial cells. Nevertheless, more sensitive and quantitative criteria for transformation of epithelial cells (perhaps biochemical) are required.

Morphologic and malignant transformations of mass cultures of rat liver epithelial cells have now been demonstrated in several laboratories.[10,12,13,16,17] A variety of carcinogens were employed. The major disadvantage of this system, in addition to the problem of scoring for transformation, is that, in general, there is a long lag (from 3 to 226 weeks) between exposure of the cells to the carcinogen and the time that one can demonstrate malignant transformation. For this reason, the epithelial system is currently not applicable for the large-scale bioassay of carcinogens.

A limitation of the cell-culture systems is that the cells may fail to activate certain drugs to the carcinogenic form. This may reflect differences between species, differences between cell types, or loss of specific drug-metabolizing enzymes during in vitro cultivation. Current approaches to this problem include the development of a wider variety of cell culture lines, addition to the culture system of microsomes from normal tissues, or the use of mixtures of "metabolizer cells" and "indicator cells." Evans, DiPaolo and their colleagues[5] have utilized a two-stage system; first the carcinogen is administered to a pregnant hamster to allow in vivo metabolism, and then the embryos are removed and their cells placed in culture and scored for transformation. These authors have demonstrated that certain known carcinogens that do not transform cells directly in culture induce transformation in this two-step assay.

Cell-culture systems may also provide assays for drugs that act as promoting agents or cofactors in the process of carcinogenesis. Sivak and Van Duuren[14,15] have developed a culture system containing a mixture of SV40-transformed 3T3 cells with a large excess of contact-inhibited 3T3 cells. Addition of the promoting agent phorbol ester enhances the outgrowth of the transformed cell population. The authors have found a good correlation between the potency of compounds as promoting agents on mouse skin and their activity in this novel assay system. There is a need to develop additional cell-culture systems that can be used to assay the effects of other promoting agents, hormonal agents, growth factors, viral agents, and other cofactors that may be involved in chemical carcinogenesis.

The use of organ cultures has the advantage that the normal geometry of complex tissues is preserved. Criteria for transformation which are similar to those used in vivo, such as hyperplasia, dysplasia, and invasiveness, can be applied in these systems, but not in dispersed-cell cultures. Cells in organ culture are also more likely to preserve a normal state of differentiation. At the current time, however, the organ-culture systems have limitations that prevent their use in the routine testing of drugs for carcinogenic activity: (1) transformation must be scored on the basis of morphology and lacks quantitative end points; (2) for the most part, there has been a failure to demonstrate that organ cultures modified by chemical carcinogens were actually tumorigenic when reimplanted into host animals, with a possible exception to this recently reported by Dao and Sinha;[4] (3) it is difficult to maintain viable organ cultures for more than one to four weeks. A promising advance is the recent finding by Dr. Bernard Lane (personal communication) that rat tracheal segments can be maintained in organ culture for at least six months.

The ultimate value of the cell-culture systems in a bioassay for carcinogens must be judged in terms of their predictive index, particularly as this relates to carcinogens in man. We strongly recommend that extensive and coordinated studies be launched to determine the validity of the hamster embryo and mouse fibroblast systems as components of one of a group of screening procedures for carcinogens. The list of carcinogenic reference compounds currently being assembled by the National Cancer Institute should be tested in these cell culture systems, and the results correlated with those obtained in whole-animal and other assays. Positive results for morphologic transformation in culture *must* be verified by assays for tumorigenicity. At the same time, there is an urgent need to develop cell-culture transformation systems that enhance the likelihood of drug metabolism as well as systems that employ epithelial cells, preferably of human origin. As these improved culture systems become available, they should be evaluated in the screening system described above.

Finally, in our enthusiasm to apply the cell-culture systems to the bioassay of carcinogens, our expectations should be modest, and the occurrence of false positives or false negatives should not lead us immediately to discredit these systems. All of the bioassays for carcinogens are models of the process in man. Some of these models are beautiful, others are less attractive, and none of them will show complete fidelity.

REFERENCES

1. Berwald, Y. and Sachs, L., *In vitro* transformation of normal cells to tumor cells by carcinogenic hydrocarbons, *J. Natl. Cancer Inst.,* 35, 641, 1965.

2. Bertram, J. S. and Heidelberger, C., Cell-cycle dependency of chemical oncogenic transformation in culture, *Proc. Am. Assoc. Cancer Res.,* 14, 70, 1973.

3. Chen, T. T. and Heidelberger, C., Quantitative studies on the malignant transformation of mouse prostate cells by carcinogenic hydrocarbons *in vitro, Int. J. Cancer,* 4, 166, 1969.

4. Dao, T. L. and Sinha, D., Mammary adenocarcinoma induced in organ culture by 7,12-dimethylbenz[*a*]anthracene, *J. Natl. Cancer Inst.,* 49, 591, 1972.

5. DiPaolo, J. A., Nelson, R. L., Donovan, P. J., and Evans, C. H., Host-mediated *in vivo-in vitro* assay for chemical carcinogenesis, *Arch. Pathol.,* 95, 380, 1973.

6. DiPaolo, J. A., Takano, K., and Popescu, N. C., Quantitation of chemically induced neoplastic transformation of Balb/3T3 cloned cell lines, *Cancer Res.,* 32, 2686, 1972.

7. DiPaolo, J. A., Donovan, P. J., and Nelson, R. L., Quantitative studies of *in vitro* transformation by chemical carcinogens, *J. Natl. Cancer Inst.,* 42, 867, 1969.

8. Freeman, A. E., Price, P. J., Igel, H. J., Maryak, J. M., and Huebner, R. J., Morphologic transformation of rat embryo cells induced by diethylnitrosamine and murine leukemia viruses, *J. Natl. Cancer Inst.,* 44, 65, 1970.

9. Freeman, A. E., Weisburger, E. K., Weisburger, J. H., Wolford, R. G., Maryak, J. M., and Huebner, R., Transformation of cell cultures as an indication of the carcinogenic potential of chemicals, *J. Natl. Cancer Inst.,* 51, 799, 1973.

10. Katsuta, H. and Takaoka, T., Carcinogenesis in tissue culture. XII. Transformation in culture of rat liver cells with 4-nitroquinoline-1-oxide, *Proceedings of the 27th General Meeting of the Japanese Cancer Association,* Tokyo, 1968, 95.

11. Marquardt, H., Kuroki, T., Huberman, E., Selkirk, J. K., Heidelberger, C., Grover, P. L., and Sims, P., Malignant transformation of cells derived from mouse prostate by epoxides and other derivatives of polycyclic hydrocarbons, *Cancer Res.,* 32, 716, 1972.

12. Namba, M., Masuji, H., and Sato, J., Carcinogenesis in tissue culture. IX. Malignant transformation of cultured rat cells treated with 4-nitroquinoline-1-oxide, *Jap. J. Exp. Med.,* 39, 253, 1969.

13. Sato, J. and Yabe, T., Carcinogenesis in tissue culture. V. Effect of long-term addition of 4-dimethylaminoazobenzene and 3-methyl-4-dimethylaminoazobenzene on liver cells in culture, *Jap. J. Exp. Med.,* 35, 445, 1965.

14. Sivak, A. and Van Duuren, B. L., Phenotypic expression of transformation: Induction in cell culture by phorbol ester, *Science,* 157, 1433, 1967.

15. Sivak, A. and Van Duuren, B. L., A cell culture system for the assessment of tumor promoting activity, *J. Natl. Cancer Inst.,* 44, 1091, 1970.

16. Weinstein, I. B., Gebert, R., Stadler, U. C., Orenstein, J. M., and Axel, R., Type C virus from cell cultures of chemically induced rat hepatomas, *Science,* 178, 1098, 1972.

17. Williams, G. M., Elliott, J. M., and Weisburger, J. H., Carcinoma after malignant conversion *in vitro* of epithelial-like cells from rat liver following exposure to chemical carcinogens, *Cancer Res.,* 33, 606, 1973.

SECTION 19
REPORT OF DISCUSSION GROUP NO. 14
CRITERIA OF NEOPLASTIC TRANSFORMATION

Henry C. Pitot

I. CRITERIA OF THE NEOPLASTIC TRANSFORMATION IN VIVO

A. Cytologic Characteristics

The histopathologic criteria for neoplasia, as currently accepted today by pathologists throughout the world, are the result of more than 100 years of study of all the variations of human neoplasia in vivo. A number of the cytologic characteristics that are utilized in these diagnoses are listed as follows: dysplasia, anaplasia, hyperplasia, nuclear-cytoplasmic ratio, cytoplasmic basophilia, mitotic aberrations, cellular and organelle polarity, and "degree of differentiation." These characteristics are all subjective, and the diagnosis of malignancy is a composite of them.

B. Biologic Criteria

1. A significant number of neoplasms, usually benign, possess a distinct capsule. Behavioristically, malignant neoplasms show varying degrees of invasiveness and growth into adjacent tissues without encapsulation. The ultimate potential of the malignant neoplasm is the metastatic or secondary growth.

2. A significant number of malignant neoplasms are aneuploid, although at very early stages of their existence many can be shown to be euploid. In the natural history of the malignant neoplasm, the degree of aneuploidy usually increases, a phenomenon associated with more rapid growth and tumor "progression." The more rapid growth of aneuploid cells is a self-selection of the "fittest."

3. Immunologic distinctions in vivo. Tumor-specific transplantation antigens are known to occur in virtually every neoplasm in vivo. In general, slowly growing spontaneous tumors are weakly antigenic, whereas rapidly growing metastasizing neoplasms demonstrate good antigenicity. A number of neoplasms in the human also exhibit embryonic antigens, a characteristic thought to be unique to neoplasms until recently.

II. CRITERIA OF THE NEOPLASTIC TRANSFORMATION IN VITRO

A. "Accepted" Characteristics of Cells Transformed in Culture

Within the last decade, conversion of normal cells growing in tissue culture to neoplastic cells in culture has been accomplished in many laboratories. The difficulty still paramount in all of these investigations is the actual determination that a cell is "transformed" from the normal to the neoplastic state. A number of laboratories have proposed criteria for this transformation. The more important of these criteria are listed as follows:

1. Production of biologically malignant neoplasms in vivo by inoculation of 10^6 or less cells into syngeneic hosts, in the absence of neoplasms produced by inoculation of comparable numbers of cells not treated with the "transforming" agent. Some "transformed" cell lines do not conform to this criterion, and some embryonic cells injected into immunosuppressed or syngeneic hosts will grow to the size of a gross tumor. The time of growth in the syngeneic host of transformed cells to detectable size may vary tremendously.

2. "Immortality" of transformed cells in culture. This is characteristic of almost all biologically neoplastic cells, although in some instances those having "immortality" in vitro do not give rise to tumors in vivo.

3. Growth of transformed cells in soft agar. With the exception of some mouse cell strains, e.g., Heidelberger's strain C3H/10T½ and transformed mouse prostate cells, transformed cells exhibiting this characteristic also produce neoplasms on inoculation into a suitable host. On the other hand, a number of biologically neoplastic tissues grown in vivo will not grow in soft agar in culture.

4. Colonies of transformed cells exhibit different morphologic and growth characteristics

in culture as compared with normal cells grown in culture. "Non-transformed" cells grow in an "ordered" way, whereas transformed cells tend to "pile up" with crisscross patterns and a higher degree of pleomorphism. However, this criterion relates only to fibroblastic cells grown in culture. So few epithelial cells have been transformed in culture that morphological criteria of transformation have not been determined accurately.

5. Loss of "contact inhibition" of cell replication and increase in saturation density by transformed cells. Again, this characteristic appears not to hold for epithelial-cell cultures, and a significant number of non-transformed cells in culture demonstrate no contact inhibition.

6. "Transformed" cells in many, but not all, instances may be agglutinated by plant lectins. Not all cells agglutinated, however, demonstrate biologic neoplasia in vivo.

7. Cells "transformed" by chemicals or viruses in culture exhibit antigenic alterations. "Spontaneous transformants" show no antigenic alterations.

8. Transformed cells may show karyotypic changes. However, cell lines that produce no tumors in vivo may be quite aneuploid, as are many "revertants" in culture.

9. "Transformed" cells usually have a greater efficiency of cloning than non-transformed cells.

B. Relative Importance of "Accepted" Criteria of Transformation in Culture

The above listing is given in order of significance as seen by the discussion panel. Clearly, the ultimate standard of neoplastic transformation is still the malignant neoplasm growing in vivo. On the other hand, all the characteristics described above apply to transformed cells and, taken together, strongly support the concept that the transformed cell is biologically neoplastic. No single criterion as yet can mark a cell transformed in culture as biologically neoplastic.

It is clear that much more work must be carried out before the scoring of cells transformed in culture can be equated totally and without reservation to a change from the normal to the neoplastic state. Virtually all of the above criteria for the in-culture transformation of cells have been established in fibroblast cultures. Very few, if any, are known to be relevant to epithelial cells in culture, which in turn are probably related to carcinomas in vivo. The latter neoplasm is by far the most common type of malignancy in the human.

RECOMMENDATIONS

The Discussion Group recommends the following:

1. The ultimate standard of the malignant transformation should still be the malignant neoplasm growing in vivo and exhibiting lethal potential for the host.

2. To date, no single criterion can be utilized to insure absolutely that cells "transformed" in vitro are biologically neoplastic. On the other hand, certain characteristics are much more relevant to the neoplastic transformation than others, as shown by experimental evidence. Much more work concerning the characteristics of the cell transformed in culture and its relationship and ultimate equating to the biologically malignant cell in vivo is absolutely necessary.

3. If cell-culture systems are utilized in the determination of carcinogenic potentiality of chemical, physical, and biological agents, the majority of the above-named criteria should be satisfied, including the first two, before definitive conclusions are made.

REFERENCES

1. Freeman, A. E. and Heubner, R. J., Problems in interpretation of experimental evidence of cell transformation, *J. Natl. Cancer Inst.*, 50, 303, 1973.
2. Rabinowitz, Z. and Sachs, L., The formation of variants with a reversion of properties of transformed cells. V. Reversion to a limited life span, *Int. J. Cancer*, 6, 388, 1970.
3. Katsuta, H. and Takaoka, T., Parameters for malignant transformation of mammalian cells treated with chemical carcinogens in tissue culture, in *Topics in Chemical Carcinogenesis*, Nakahara, W., Takayama, S., Sugimura, T., and Odashima, S., Eds., University of Tokyo Press, 1972, 389.
4. Heidelberger, C., Chemical oncogenesis in culture, *Adv. Cancer Res.*, 18, 317, 1973.

SECTION 20
REPORT OF DISCUSSION GROUP NO. 15
PROBLEMS OF DEVELOPMENT OF SYSTEMS
WITH MATERIALS OF HUMAN ORIGIN

Aaron Freeman

INTRODUCTION

The present methods of testing the carcinogenic activity of chemicals depend on testing these compounds in animal-model systems and extrapolating the results to predict the effects of the same agents in man. Such an interpretation may be unwarranted and, indeed, may even be dangerous. Human cell-culture systems have already proved to be useful in assessing in vivo results in other areas of biomedical research, particularly in cytogenetics and in the isolation, identification, and characterization of human viruses. Thus, if responsive human cell cultures were available, it probably would be preferable to use these models to evaluate agents that are potentially carcinogenic for man.

EFFECTS OF CARCINOGENS
IN CELL CULTURES

Dr. Leonard Hayflick reported that the human diploid embryonic lung cell strain (WI-38) was not transformed by single or multiple treatments with polycyclic hydrocarbons. Further, negative transforming results were also obtained in similar testing of cell strains derived from whole human embryos, Down's syndrome, or xeroderma pigmentosum. Dr. Hayflick did find, however, that human cells could be used to measure the toxic effects of chemicals.

Dr. Howard Igel presented similar negative findings with more than 50 cell strains derived from normal, benign, or malignant source material. However, he did present the following evidence for urethane-induced transformation of two cell strains derived from neurofibrosarcomas of siblings affected with von Recklinghausen's disease. Starting with contact-inhibited diploid-cell cultures with normal karyotype and limited life span in culture, he obtained appearance of morphologically altered foci in multiple urethane-treated samples in each of five experiments. It was difficult to develop continuous cell lines from the morpho-

logically altered foci; however, such continuous cell lines were obtained from several individual foci. These rapidly growing cultures were subpassaged for more than 150 population doublings; they are heteroploid and induce tumors in X-irradiated mice. Von Recklinghausen's disease is genetically inherited, and these patients are at extreme high risk for the development of benign neurofibromas, which then tend to convert spontaneously in situ to malignant neurofibrosarcomas. Thus, cell lines derived from these patients may also be genetically predisposed to cell transformation in vitro.

Dr. Paul Price reported that he had attempted to establish continuous cell lines from more than 150 assorted human tumors. He initiated cell growth from virtually every tumor, but only in five cases was he able to develop a continuous cell line with characteristics of tumor cells. Most cell strains derived from human tumor appeared to consist of diploid cells. In subsequent discussion, Dr. Freeman suggested that if continuous cell lines can be established only rarely from human tumors, then for the same reasons, it may be equally difficult to develop a continuous transformed-cell line once morphological transformation is observed.

Dr. Leila Diamond presented a view on the metabolism of carcinogens. It is generally accepted that most chemicals have to be metabolized to active forms before they become carcinogenic. Thus, in order to achieve transformation, either the active form must be used or the cell must possess the necessary enzyme systems for making the conversion. At the present time, only the metabolism of hydrocarbons has been studied to any extent. The microsomal enzyme aryl hydrocarbon hydroxylase (AHH) is probably involved in the conversion of hydrocarbons to more carcinogenic forms, which may be epoxides. In general, these facts have been demonstrated: (1) primary rodent cell cultures have AHH activity; (2) there is a strong correlation between AHH activity and transformation of rodent cells in culture; (3)

human embryo cells show AHH activity in primary culture, but lose this activity after a few passages and become more resistant to the toxic effects of hydrocarbons; (4) there is a wide variation of AHH activity between human embryos; and (5) primary human epithelial cells have higher AHH activity than fibroblasts. Dr. Diamond also presented a number of suggestions regarding the selection of human cell cultures appropriate for transformation studies. These comments will be included in a subsequent section of this report.

Dr. Richard Kouri spoke about his screening of whole human embryo cultures for AHH activity. Cultured human cells possess levels of AHH ranging from non-detectable to about those of mouse or rat cells. He suggested that a significant part of the negative reports concerning the transformability of human cells in culture probably results from these very low levels of activating enzymes, and that a screening test for detecting human cell lines that possess higher AHH levels should precede any large-scale attempt to transform these cells by polycyclic aromatic hydrocarbon carcinogens.

Dr. T. Timothy Crocker presented comparative data on the effects of benzo[a]pyrene on tracheal-organ cultures of hamster, fetal human, and adult human origin. After 7 to 18 days in organ culture, benzo[a]pyrene, at a concentration of 10 μg per ml of culture medium, produced epithelial hyperplasia in hamster and fetal human trachea. Thus, the same dose produced the same type of lesion in both systems. However, benzo[a]pyrene did not induce hyperplasia in adult tracheal organ cultures. Dr. Crocker also presented a detailed report regarding some of the technical problems related to developing organ-cell cultures of human origin.

Dr. Bernard Lane was able to maintain living, fully ciliated rat trachea in vitro for periods up to six months. His method depended on sharp incision and production of uniform tracheal rings, which floated in the medium. These cells were incubated in CO_2, and special effort was made to prevent high oxygen levels. Benzo[a]pyrene caused hyperplasia of the epithelium surrounding these tracheal rings. There was no invasion of the basal membrane, but the epithelial cells did appear to be atypical. No cell-culture or tumor-inducing experiments were carried out to confirm whether these atypical epithelial cells have other characteristics of malignant cells.

RESEARCH-RELATED QUESTIONS AND PROBLEMS

The Committee listed a series of questions and problems, all worthy of extensive investigation. The following list is included without comment. Selected areas of special interest will be identified and discussed (see Recommendations).

A. Factors affecting selection of the human donor cell or organ culture
  1. Genetic background of the donor
    a. Predisposition to cancer
    b. Metabolism of potentially carcinogenic compounds
    c. Sex
    d. Age
  2. Virus profile
    a. Infectious agents
    b. Latent agents
  3. Treatment prior to cell-culture processing (especially in regard to previous drug therapy)
  4. Types of cells
    a. Epithelial versus fibroblastic
    b. Differentiated versus undifferentiated
    c. Specific organ versus whole embryo
  5. Normal versus malignant origin of cells
  6. Age of the cells in culture
    a. Metabolic time
    b. Population-doubling level
B. Culture conditions
  1. Media
  2. Serum species
  3. Inactivation of a carcinogen by the medium or by other factors
  4. Type of exposure to a chemical (single dose versus repeated doses)
  5. Growth phase of cells during exposure to a chemical
C. What characteristics will be accepted as reasonable evidence of transformation?
D. How do we test for tumorigenicity of the transformed cells?
E. What does a negative test mean?
F. Do our present cultures contain the target cell?
G. How do we obtain enough of the desired human material?
H. How do we resolve the legal and moral considerations involved in obtaining and using human cell sources?
I. Human material is not available from strictly

inbred colonies, but it is available from groups with a higher-than-usual frequency of inbreeding.

J. What is the validity of using in vitro tests to predict in vivo activity?

RECOMMENDATIONS

1. A major effort should be made to develop human organ-culture methods for testing the effects of carcinogens. Organ cultures present an intact cell population, theoretically containing the target cells in association with their accustomed surrounding cell population. We suggest the use of organ slices in the initial efforts, but do not discount the development of whole-organ-culture systems. A combination of organ- and cell-culture techniques would allow an initial exposure to chemicals under organ-culture conditions, followed by dispersion into monolayer cultures for the isolation and characterization of the transformed cells.

2. Transformation studies should be carried out in monolayer cultures of epithelioid as well as of fibroblastic cell populations. Primary cultures of kidney, liver, skin, and amnion can be used for initial studies. Basic research is needed for the development of human diploid epithelial-cell lines.

3. Metabolism of chemicals other than the polycyclic hydrocarbons must be studied. Cell banks of cultures known to have specific metabolic activating systems should be established. As an initial project, it would be worthwhile to study the transformability of a series of primary whole human embryo cultures (still containing an epithelial component) that have been characterized at least with regard to AHH activity.

4. The role of chemicals and viruses as activating or promoting agents should be studied.

5. For drug evaluation, cells should be as close to normal as possible. However, in view of the apparent difficulty in demonstrating chemically induced transformation in human-cell cultures, continuous cell lines or cell strains with a controlled element of abnormal characteristics may have to be used.

6. The demonstration of the tumorigenicity of a human cell is virtually impossible as an autograft; as an allograft, it is complicated by moral, ethical, legal, and immunological problems. Thus, evidence of tumor induction as a xenograft in, for example, nude or ALS-treated mice should probably be accepted as an indication of the tumorigenic potential of the transformed cells. The tumors produced must, however, be confirmed with respect to their malignant pathology and species of origin.

7. A committee should be established to procure and provide human material for cell and organ cultures, and to establish guidelines to cope with the existing medicolegal and ethical complications that hinder collection of human material. This same committee might also concern itself with obtaining material from known inbred human populations, particularly those that may exhibit a genetic predisposition to cancer.

SECTION 21
SUMMARY AND CONCLUDING REMARKS

David P. Rall

In a brief presentation, I would like to point out some of the salient points, both explicit and implicit, in this Conference, and, in so doing, I hope to sharpen our focus on one or two of the problems. First, I think, it might be wise for all to remember that the first Food and Drug crisis was caused by an elixir of sulfanilamide and that the laboratory tests necessary to demonstrate that this was the problem took a day or two. The second crisis was caused by thalidomide. Those not convinced by the effects on rabbits would have had to wait for monkey tests, and the resolution would have taken weeks to months.

The question, I think, we are facing at this Conference is this: "It there now a third Food and Drug crisis, namely carcinogenesis and carcinogenesis testing, which apparently will take two to three years to resolve?" We have, in the course of this Conference, learned a great deal about species differences in drug disposition and metabolism, about strain and species differences in animals highly resistant and highly sensitive to carcinogens, about problems of extrapolation of laboratory animal data to man, of dose problems and time problems, and of probability and statistical problems.

In looking at the carcinogenesis problem, it is important to recognize that a positive response to a carcinogen is modified by at least three separate factors: The first is the innate susceptibility of the animal, including perhaps viral and genetic backgrounds. The second is the innate drug metabolism and disposition apparatus. It seems to me that the metabolic activation of carcinogens can be basically regarded as the first step in the disposition of these compounds. This innate apparatus appears to be largely genetically controlled. It differs very widely from species to species, and I think we should remember that, for some drugs, it has been shown that it differs almost as much within the human species as it does among the various other mammals. I think this underlines an urgent need for extensive studies of human pharmacology in the first patients studied. These should involve more than just one or two or three patients; eventually the number should extend to as many

as 30 or 40 subjects. Third, environmental conditions are also important; they can affect not only innate susceptibility but also drug disposition. Of some of these conditions we are all aware: the gastrointestinal-tract flora; the diet; other drugs; and a whole variety of environmental exposures. And, as we try to understand the meaning of studies in laboratory animals and their relevance to man, I think we must keep in mind each of those three factors: the innate susceptibility, the drug metabolism and disposition apparatus, and environmental conditions. For instance, there was considerable discussion of the need for positive controls, and basically, I might say, I agree with Dr. Price on this because of the possible genetic and environmental or dietary changes in any one laboratory over a period of a few years. It would seem to me that at least *occasional* use of a positive control in a laboratory would be necessary, not for each study, but perhaps every two or three years.

In terms of the statistical treatment of carcinogenesis data, I think we have a long way to go. It seems clear to me that the use of the t-test and of the significance of differences in incidence of tumors is no longer a very useful or relevant tool, and I think we must develop new statistical methods to answer questions of relative risks with some sort of probability level. This was not discussed as much as I would have liked.

The rapid presumptive tests that were presented here are, I think, of major importance. No single test seems to be ideal, and I'm sure that none will ever be. I would like to applaud the National Cancer Institute for its approach of prospective study, using, I think, 85 compounds known to be positive or negative in long-term rodent tests, and for beginning to assemble this data base. A careful comparison of the results, first in the classic test and then in the new rapid test, should go a long way to demonstrate the validity or the lack of validity of these tests.

Also, the clues presented by Dr. Fraumeni and his drug studies must be very carefully explored. Here is an instance known to have caused a positive reaction in man. Do animal bioassay studies, either the classic long-term or the current short-term studies, predict what we now know are positive human responses? I think that answers to this question will be very important.

Let me return now to the problem of new-drug development and carcinogenicity. For rapidly manifest drug effects, animal studies have greater relevance during Phase I in the very early clinical trial, and again primarily for the first few patients. As clinical experience is developed, it becomes more and more evident that "the proper study of mankind is man," but for *delayed* effects, carcinogenicity in particular, this is not true. We must base our evaluations on experimental studies. Human epidemiology is vital and we certainly must do more of it, but it cannot help us in early studies; the lag period of 10 to 20 years is simply too long.

In the world of drug development, one must deal with such organizations as the Food and Drug Administration, with the pharmaceutical industry, and with an increasing variety of interested parties. Currently, a potential new drug may be tested in man cautiously and under careful and, I think, excellent clinical supervision; this, I think, is important. After acute and fairly short-term toxicity tests in a few species of laboratory animals, assuming the drug has therapeutic potential, it is then studied in more and more patients; long-term animal studies are started, so that the chronic-toxicity studies will be completed before a large number of patients have been exposed. This general plan is now being challenged. We now have heard requests to perform the long-term chronic life-time carcinogenicity studies before clinical testing is initiated. It is claimed that this would decrease the risk to the patients in the early clinical trial and provide us with safe and more effective drugs. I am not at all sure that this is true, and I think we must examine this concept. The introduction of any drug in demand entails risks, potential hazards, not only for the *first* person receiving that drug, but really for *all* subsequent patients who receive it. Although we know quite a bit about the full clinical potential of a drug by the time it is marketed, for most drugs on the market today there is *some* hazard in their administration to *some* segment of the population. We all know that aspirin, penicillin, and so forth, carry with them some risks, however low, when administered to a patient. What I'm saying, therefore, is that risks with drugs are always with us.

This great public concern over drug hazards, I think, comes from a sort of expectation of perfection, engendered within the United States population by such magazines as the *Reader's Digest* in their wonderful articles of supertherapeutics a few decades ago. It seems there was always a miracle cure for this or that or the other disease. The benefits were headlined, the risks ignored, and I think the American public was badly informed.

The question, then, is this: "What is the harm in delaying Phase I in the initial clinical experiment for the two-year carcinogenicity studies?" I think that the major problem is the lack of follow-through, of continuity in the progress of the drug-development process. It seems to me — and I'm not sure this is widely recognized — that the development of a new drug is a surprisingly fragile process. Trivial reasons can abort an apparently promising lead, and I am convinced that to impose a two- to three-year delay in the critical midperiod of the development of a new drug would most seriously impede the entire drug-development process.

Now, what can we do? It is clear from all we have heard in reports and discussions at this Conference that animal tests for carcinogenicity are hardly cut and dried. There really is notable lack of agreement on what tests and what species to use, how the tests should be performed, and so forth. We are all, I think, aware that the standard two-year mouse and rat tests will give us both false positives and false negatives. We all know that the scientific community is very diverse and heterogeneous. It contains among absolutely reputable and dedicated scientists those, on the one hand, who feel that any risk of neoplasia is an absolute black mark for any compound, and those, on the other hand, who feel that the only true carcinogens are those that have been proved by epidemiological studies on man. It seems to me, therefore, that any Federal regulatory decision or policy in this area can be — and in today's climate certainly will be — challenged, and the challenge will be buttressed by a certain amount of reputable scientific opinion. Such decisions, however, are necessary, and in the face of disagreement among the experts — the scientists — final approval or ratification of the decision must, I think, come from the public sector of society in general. I think this is proper; it demands, however, that renewed efforts be made to educate and inform the public. People must not expect perfection in drugs in what is clearly an imperfect world. Such education will be difficult, but I think it is necessary.

Let me spell out, briefly, the nature of the carcinogenicity testing that I feel is necessary and proper during development of a new drug. We say at the outset that life-time studies, though not necessarily life-time feeding, are mandatory for a compound that is to be marketed. Such studies are not perfect, but the need to protect the public demands them for all marketed drugs. At the other end of the drug-development process, I think we can do more than we have been doing, and I would particularly use rapid tests as they become perfected and validated.

I believe is it important that as many new compounds as possible get tested in man, and I would look forward to the development of the research I.N.D. concept, which I hope will allow this. A limited number of patients would be studied under highly controlled conditions after limited, but adequate, toxicity studies. These studies would include standard tests for acute and subacute toxicity; they would consider structure—activity relationships to see if the compound under investigation was related to known carcinogens; and they would include a battery of the new presumptive tests. If any of these studies indicated that there was reason to believe the compound might be carcinogenic, then, I think, a two-year study probably would be necessary. If, however, none of these studies — standard brief toxicity studies, presumptive tests, or consideration of the structure—activity relationships — suggested that carcinogenicity would be a problem, then, I would think, it would be safe to move forward into an initial clinical trial. Clinical pharmacology, pharmacokinetics, and metabolism must be emphasized in these early studies. Let me emphasize what has been said before: these studies must include, on the part of the patients, informed consent that is *truly* informed consent. It would seem to me, then, that after these patients had been studied, one could move on to the further development of the drug in much the way used now. In terms of the specific research needs in this area, I think these are obvious and need continued and intensified development of foreshortened tests. We also need considerably more public information and education in pharmacology and toxicology. In addition, there is an area to which I have devoted little time, but which, I think, is of utmost importance, and that is the need to develop our human epidemiology resources much more actively than we have. We need a national death index, and clearly, we also need an adverse-drug-reaction surveillance system on a scale that covers perhaps up to 200,000 or 300,000 patients, and a record-linkage system that will allow us to link the drugs that patients received with the diagnosis and the disease that eventually will develop. That is a tall order, but I think we can do it.

SECTION 22
RECOMMENDATIONS OF THE CONFERENCE AS STATED BY THE CONFERENCE CHAIRMAN

Leon Golberg

The Conference was intended to serve as a springboard for action. Many valuable suggestions were put forward and many inportant conclusions were reached in the course of the formal presentations, discussion group reports, panel discussions, and summation by the panel on "Strategy of Carcinogenesis Testing in the Plan of Development of New Drugs." In order to ensure that these ideas are not overlooked, and to facilitate implementation of worthwhile proposals, a general review of the recommendations is presented below. It should be stressed that neither official sanction nor approval has been sought for these suggestions. It would hardly be surprising to find that many experts take issue with one or more of these recommendations. Nevertheless, a sincere effort has been made to reflect the opinion of the majority of specialists on each topic, in the hope that their conclusions may be helpful to the reader.

PRESENT STATUS OF ESTABLISHED PROCEDURES

The report of the Panel on Carcinogenesis of the FDA Advisory Committee on Protocols for Safety Evaluation (see Section 9) has specified conditions for the conduct of life-span studies intended to assess the carcinogenic potential of test compounds. A number of issues remain unresolved, however, or are still the subject of debate. One of these is the number of species and the nature of the species to be used.

In practice, time is often a more crucial factor than cost when the carcinogenic potential of a drug is under investigation. The predominant need is for an unequivocal "yes" or "no" answer to the question of carcinogenesis, even though it is accepted that no test or tests can totally exclude the possibility that a drug possesses the potential to induce neoplasia. From the standpoint of this need, the use of mice as well as of rats has the merit of increasing the assurance of safety, but at a greater risk of yielding observations whose interpretation is a matter of opinion among pathol-

ogists or a source of contention among statisticians. There is a case for using F_1 hybrids of genetically stable inbred strains of mice, but as far as rats are concerned, the established outbred strains will doubtless continued to be used. The BD rat strains, painstakingly developed by Prof. H. Druckrey, are worthy of much greater attention than they have received so far in this country.

The need for standardization and use of semi-synthetic diets becomes ever more compelling with the growth of our awareness of incidental contaminants in commercial chow diets.

Selection of the highest dose of test compound to be used in the study is the most crucial decision of the entire investigation. In recommending the use of the "highest possible dose that will permit valid interpretation of the experimental observations," the report of the Discussion Group concerned with this problem (see Section 4) has taken pains to elaborate some of the important considerations that pertain to the determination of this dose.

The inception of a carcinogenesis test should involve exposure of the developing fetus to the drug *in utero* as well as continuous postnatal administration of the compound for a finite period, 18 months in mice and two years in rats. Any requirement for more extended periods of exposure and/or observation is likely to be incompatible with the necessary freedom to choose appropriate strains of animals and with survival of an adequate proportion of such animals.

On the difficult subject of the use of positive controls, the choice whether or not to include animals treated with known carcinogens should remain optional. For the purpose of testing new drugs, it is likely that, in most instances, sound practical considerations will dictate a decision not to use positive controls.

Turning from the conduct of tests to the question of interpretation of the results, it is first necessary for each laboratory engaged in studies of this sort to ascertain the incidence of spontaneous tumors in the strains of animals under the conditions used. A constantly updated record of the frequency and nature of the spontaneous tumors observed in untreated controls provides a valuable background against which to judge current results. The classification of tumors, and particularly the diagnosis of malignancy, is a continuing problem, to which more intensive and systematic effort should be devoted, particularly by pathologists, not statisticians.

SHORT-TERM PREDICTIVE TESTS

This area of research not only merits encouragement and support, but is also likely to yield the greatest advances and benefits in return for the funds expended.

Assessment of DNA damage anu repair synthesis brought about in vitro or in a combined in vivo/in vitro system holds great promise as a bioassay for carcinogens. The potential utility, for carcinogen-screening purposes, of tests for genetic damage is worthy of further exploration. In all instances, the tests referred to should be carried out not only with the test compound, but also with its metabolically activated products. Procedures for bringing about such activation in vitro are available and should be integrated into each test where activation of the compound is necessary.

Cell- and organ-culture systems appropriate for study of the action of carcinogens have been developed to a satisfactory degree, but the need for epithelial-cell systems still exists. Understanding of the criteria of neoplastic transformation, and of the nature and sources of artifacts in such tests, has progressed to a point where it is possible to insist that the majority of the criteria shall have been checked before definitive conclusions are drawn. A combined host-mediated tissue-culture technique probably represents the most advanced procedure available at present in this field of research.

Ideally, the development of systems employing cells, tissues, and organs of human origin should provide screening procedures whose results would be directly applicable to the assessment of hazard to man. Many problems, not all of them scientific, have to be resolved before suitable procedures can be developed. Nevertheless, there is need to persevere in the pursuit of these worthwhile objectives.

INDEX

A

2-AAF, *see* 2-Acetylaminofluorene
N-Acetoxyacetylaminofluorene,
  levels of DNA repair synthesis in xeroderma pigmento-
    sum, 87
N-Acetoxy-2-acetylaminofluorene,
  induction of single-strand breaks in hepatic DNA, 96
2-Acetylaminofluorene,
  carcinogenic activity, 81
  evaluation of tumorigenicity, 11
  induction of single-strand breaks in hepatic DNA, 96
  tumor development, dietary inhibition, 17
1-Acetyl-1-isonicotinioylhydrazine,
  carcinogenicity in mice, 48
Acinar-cell adenomas, pancreatic,
  incidence in CRCD control rats, 8
  spontaneous development in CRCD control rats, 6
Acridine dyes,
  effect of DNA repair, 76
Adenine phosphoribosyl transferase,
  deficiency in mutant hamster cells, 104
Adenocanthomas,
  incidence in inbred mouse strains and wild mice, 62
Adenocarcinomas,
  adrenal, 6, 7
    incidence in CRCD control rats, 7
    spontaneous development in CRCD control rats, 6
  cervical,
    relation to drug exposure, 51
  mammary, 6–9, 57
    differences in incidence between control groups of
      CRCD rats, 9
    incidence in CRCD control rats, 7, 8
    incidence in Sprague-Dawley and Fischer rats, 57
    spontaneous development in CRCD control rats, 6
  parathyroid,
    spontaneous development in CRCD control rats, 6
  pituitary, 6, 8
    incidence in CRCD control rats, 8
    spontaneous development in CRCD control rats, 6
  pulmonary,
    description, 72
  salivary-gland, 6, 7
    incidence in CRCD control rats, 7
    spontaneous development in CRCD control rats, 6
  thyroid, 6, 8
    incidence in CRCD control rats, 8
    spontaneous development in CRCD control rats, 6
  uterine, 6, 7, 63
    incidence in CRCD control rats, 7
    incidence in inbred mouse strains, 63
    spontaneous development in CRCD control rats, 6
  vaginal,
    relation to drug exposure, 51
Adenofibromas, *see* Fibroadenomas
Adenomas,
  acinar-cell, pancreatic, 6, 8
    incidence in CRCD control rats, 8

    spontaneous development in CRCD control rats, 6
  adrenal, 6, 7
    incidence in CRCD control rats, 7
    spontaneous development in CRCD control rats, 6
  adrenal cortical, 8, 57, 60
    incidence in CRCD control rats, 8
    incidence in inbred mouse strains, 60
    incidence in Sprague-Dawley and Fischer rats, 57
  apocrine,
    incidence in Sprague-Dawley and Fischer rats, 57
  bronchial,
    incidence in Sprague-Dawley and Fischer rats, 58
  cutaneous,
    incidence in CRCD control rats, 8
  hepatic, 6, 7
    incidence in CRCD control rats, 7
    spontaneous development in CRCD control rats, 6
  hepatocellular,
    incidence in CRCD control rats, 8
  islet-cell,
    incidence in CRCD control rats, 8
  mammary, 6–8, 57
    incidence in CRCD control rats, 7, 8
    incidence in Sprague-Dawley and Fischer rats, 57
    spontaneous development in CRCD control rats, 6
  ovarian, tubular,
    incidence in inbred mouse strains, 62
  pancreatic,
    spontaneous development in CRCD control rats, 6
  parathyroid,
    spontaneous development in CRCD control rats, 6
  pituitary, 6–9, 57, 60
    differences in incidence between control groups of
      CRCD rats, 9
    incidence in CRCD control rats, 7, 8
    incidence in inbred mouse strains, 60
    incidence in Sprague-Dawley and Fischer rats, 57
    spontaneous development in CRCD control rats, 6
  pulmonary, 48, 72, 82
    assay in compressed carcinogenicity tests, 82
    description, 72
    effect of isoniazid administration, 48
    effect of metronidazole administration, 48
    induction by 1-acetyl-1-isonicotinoylhydrazine in
      mice, 48
  renal,
    incidence in CRCD control rats, 8
  renal cortical, 6, 7
    incidence in CRCD control rats, 7
    spontaneous development in CRCD control rats, 6
  sebaceous,
    incidence in Sprague-Dawley and Fischer rats, 57
  thyroid, 6, 8, 57
    incidence in CRCD control rats, 8
    incidence in Sprague-Dawley and Fischer rats, 57
    spontaneous development in CRCD control rats, 6
Adenosarcomas, pancreatic,
  incidence in CRCD control rats, 7
Adrenal cortical tumors,

incidence in CRCD control rats, 8
incidence in inbred mouse strains, 60, 61, 63
incidence in Sprague-Dawley and Fischer rats, 57
incidence in wild mice, 63
Adrenal-gland tumors,
adenocarcinomas, 6, 7
incidence in CRCD control rats, 7
spontaneous development in CRCD control rats, 6
adenomas, 6, 7
incidence in CRCD control rats, 7
spontaneous development in CRCD control rats, 6
cortical adenomas, 8, 57, 60
incidence in CRCD control rats, 8
incidence in inbred mouse strains, 60
incidence in Sprague-Dawley and Fischer rats, 57
cortical carcinomas,
incidence in inbred mouse strains, 60
ganglioneuroblastomas,
incidence in Sprague-Dawley and Fischer rats, 57
pheochromocytomas, 6–9, 57, 63
differences in incidence between control groups of
CRCD rats, 9
incidence in CRCD control rats, 7, 8
incidence in inbred mouse strains, 63
incidence in Sprague-Dawley and Fischer rats, 57
incidence in wild mice, 63
spontaneous development in CRCD control rats, 6
AFB₁, *see* Aflatoxin B₁
Aflatoxin,
binding to DNA, RNA and protein, 84
toxic action, 84
tumorigenicity following prenatal exposure, 25
Aflatoxin B,
tumorigenicity following prenatal exposure, 26
Aflatoxin B₁,
alteration of toxicity by dietary lipotrope deficiency,
17
effects of dietary deficiencies on carcinogenicity, 17, 18
lipotropic nutrients, 17, 18
vitamin A, 18
induction of single-strand breaks in hepatic DNA, 96
African green monkey,
lymphoma-virus susceptibility, 67
AHH, *see* Aryl hydrocarbon hydroxylase
Alkylating agents,
carcinogenic activity, 83
carcinogenic effect in man, 52
effect on mutation in Chinese hamster cells, 104
potential to produce aplastic anemia, 53
Rosenkranz prescreening test, 102
Amines, aromatic,
association between carcinogenicity and mutagenicity,
104
classification of chemical carcinogens, 80
DNA repair, 106
metabolic activation, 106
o-Aminoazotoluene,
tumorigenicity following prenatal exposure, 26
3-Aminodibenzofuran,
carcinogenic activity, 81
2-Aminopurine nitrate,
determination of mutagenicity, 85

3-Aminotriazole,
use as positive control compound, 30, 32, 33
Androgenic-anabolic steroids,
carcinogenic effect in man, 52
Androgens, exogenous,
carcinogenic effects in man, 52
Anemia, aplastic,
carcinogenic effect of treatment with exogenous androgens, 52
leukemogenic agents, 53
Angiosarcomas, cardiorespiratory,
incidence in Sprague-Dawley and Fischer rats, 58
Animal-model systems,
extrapolation of results to man, 115
Antilymphocyte serum,
carcinogenic effect in man, 51, 52
Antimetabolites,
carcinogenic effect in man, 51, 52
Aplastic anemia,
carcinogenic effect of treatment with exogenous androgens, 52
leukemogenic agents, 53
APRT, *see* Adenine phosphoribosyl transferase
Arrhenoblastomas,
incidence in Sprague-Dawley and Fischer rats, 57
Arsenic,
carcinogenic effect in man, 51
Arsenicals, inorganic,
carcinogenic effects in man, 52
Aryl hydrocarbon hydroxylase,
activity in human cell cultures, 116
activity in rodent cell cultures, 115
conversion of hydrocarbons, 115
correlation between AAH activity and transformation
in rodent cell cultures, 115
correlation with dietary casein level, 17
effect of chow diets on activity, 17
Astrocytomas,
encephalic, 6, 7
incidence in CRCD control rats, 7
spontaneous development in CRCD control rats, 6
neural,
incidence in Sprague-Dawley and Fischer rats, 57
8-Azaguanine,
resistance in diploid human cells, 105
Azo compounds, 80
Azoethane,
tumorigenicity following prenatal exposure, 26
Azoxyethane,
tumorigenicity following prenatal exposure, 26
Azoxymethane,
tumorigenicity following prenatal exposure, 26

B

Baboon,
lymphoma-virus susceptibility, 67
B[a]P, *see* Benzo[a]pyrene
Base-pair substitutions, mutagenic, 102, 103
Basal-cell carcinomas,
incidence in CRCD control rats, 8

spontaneous development in CRCD control rats, 6
Benign tumors,
  definition, 41
  progression to malignancy, 41
  spontaneous conversion to malignancy, 115
Benzene,
  potential to produce aplastic anemia, 53
Benzo[a]pyrene,
  carcinogenic activity, 38
  carcinogenic effect on cell cultures, 86
  effect on cell cultures of animal and human origin, 116
  isolation from coal tar, 79
  tumorigenicity following prenatal exposure, 26
  tumor-initiating activity, 37
  use as positive control compound, 35, 36
Bioassay, combination, host-mediated, 93
Bladder concretions, 42, 81, 82
Bleomycin,
  induction of single-strand breaks in hepatic DNA, 96
Brain tumors,
  astrocytomas, 6, 7
    incidence in CRCD control rats, 7
    spontaneous development in CRCD control rats, 6
  gliomas, 6–8
    incidence in CRCD control rats, 7, 8
    spontaneous development in CRCD control rats, 6
  neurofibrosarcomas, 6, 7
    incidence in CRCD control rats, 7
    spontaneous development in CRCD control rats, 6
5-Bromodeoxyuridine,
  resistance in mutant hamster cells, 104
Bromouracil,
  determination of mutagenicity, 85
Butadienediepoxide,
  carcinogenic activity, 81
2(n-Butyloxycarbonylmethylene)thiazolid-4-one,
  carcinogenic activity, 81

C

Caffeine,
  determination of mutagenicity, 85
  false positive results, 102
Calcium,
  content in chow diets, 18
Calculi, urinary,
  interrelationship with neoplasms of the bladder, 47
  presence in tumorigenesis, 42
Camptothecin,
  induction of single-strand breaks in hepatic DNA, 96
Cancer therapy,
  cytotoxic agents, 52
  radioisotopes, 51
  stilbestrol, 52
Carcinogenesis,
  dose – duration relationship, 11
  effects of dietary deficiencies, 17, 18
  effect of air pollution, 35–39
  effect of tobacco smoke, 35
  induction period, 42
  inhibition by induction of increased microsomal

enzyme activity, 19
  initiation and promotion systems, 82, 83
  irreversible response, 41
  irritation by concretions, 42
  latent period, 11, 26
    dose-dependence, 11
    proportion of total life span, 11
    reduction in prenatal exposure, 26
  malignancy criteria and differentiation, 71
  mechanisms of dietary action, 18, 19
  metabolic activation, 75–78
    balance between pathways, 76
    manipulation of pathways, 78
    reactivity with cellular macromolecules, 78
  monitoring in man, 41
  neoplastic transformation, 113, 114
  one-hit hypothesis, 92
  positive controls, 35–39
  post-transplant, 52
  potential of respiratory-pollutant particulates, 35
  tests involving induction of neoplasia, 91–93
  transplacental, 23, 82, 83
    initiation and promotion systems, 82, 83
    susceptibility of offspring, 23
Carcinogenic tests,
  adverse-drug-reaction surveillance, 121
  analysis of data, 42
  basis for evaluation, 120
  clinical pharmacology studies, 121
  diets, 17–20
    casein level, 17
    chow, 17
    fats, 17
    folate deficiency, 19
    folic acid deficiency, 19
    lipotrope deficiency, 17–19
    manipulation, 20
    mechanisms of action, 18, 19
    natural-product, 17
    protein deficiency, 17, 19
    riboflavin deficiency, 17
    semisynthetic purified, 17
  dosage levels, 3, 4, 47
    vitamin A deficiency, 18
    range for hormonal carcinogens, 47
    therapeutic levels for man, 4
    WHO recommendations for highest dose, 3
  dose–response curves, 4
  dose selection and administration, 22
  drug development, 120
  duration, 5, 23–26
    guidelines for establishment, 5
    recommendations of different committees, 24, 25
  experimental design for life-span study, 1
  experimental protocol, 42
  extrapolation of animal data to man, 45–47
    assessment of statistical significance, 47
    metabolism of test compound, 46
    route of administration, 46
    selection of appropriate test animal, 45
    transplacental administration of carcinogens, 46
FDA operating policy and priorities, 43

Federal regulations, 120, 121
interpretation of results, 5–10, 41–43, 45–49
  in relation to test animals, 41–43
  in terms of significance to man, 45–49
  significance of spontaneous-tumor incidence, 5–10
licensing of toxicological laboratories, 49
maximal tolerated dose, 47
  definitions, 47
  WHO recommendations, 47
metabolism studies, 121
modification of positive response, 119
national death index, 121
outline of experiment for rodents, 2
pathology procedures, 5
pharmacokinetics studies, 121
positive controls, 10, 29–34
  active intermediates, 30
  application, 10
  compounds in current use, 31–33
  consistency of response, 34
  correlation of negative results with sensitivity of test
    system, 30
  definition, 29
  disposal of residues, 30
  evaluation of relative sensitivities of bioassay systems,
    29, 30
  interpretation of indefinite response, 29
  number of test animals, 30
  potential hazards, 10, 30
  stated purpose, 10
  use of historical background data, 10
prescreening tests, 101–106
  mutagenesis assessment, 101–106
  National Cancer Institute study, 101
  procedural characteristics, 101
present status, 123, 124
  chow diets, 123
  conditions for lifespan studies, 123
  highest possible dose, 123
  incidence of spontaneous tumors, 123, 124
  interpretation of results, 123, 124
  number and nature of species, 123
  period of drug exposure, 123
  positive controls, 123
  semisynthetic diets, 123
rapid presumptive tests, 119
record-linkage system, 121
relevance to man, 119
route of administration, 4
safety evaluation, 41–43
  analysis of data, 42
  carcinogenic potential to test animals, 41–43
  experimental protocol, 42
selection of test animals, 15
sensitivity, 26, 29, 30, 42
  degree required for carcinogenic assay, 42
  integration of prenatal exposure with long-term post-
    natal exposure, 26
  limiting factor, 42
  relative, of bioassay systems, 29, 30
short-term tests, 79–87, 91–93, 95–99, 101–106, 124
  assessment of DNA damage and repair synthesis, 124

  cell cultures, 124
  chemical-interaction measurements, 95–99
  compressed carcinogenicity tests, 82, 83
  criteria, 79, 80
  epithelial-cell systems, 124
  formazan deposition test, 81
  hyperplasia test, 81
  in vitro tests, 83–87
  in vivo tests, 80–83
  organ cultures, 124
  prediction for carcinogenicity in man, 101
  screening procedures, 124
  sebaceous-gland suppression tests, 81
  subacute toxicity test, 81
statistical considerations, 1, 3, 4, 11, 42, 43, 47, 119
  benefits of larger numbers of animals, 3
  biologic validity, 11
  comparison of tumor development in test and control
    animals, 3, 4
  correlation to biological findings, 11
  interpretation of results, 11
  "no effect" level, 4
  number of survivors, 1
  significance in extrapolation of animal data to man,
    47
  threshold dose, 42, 43
  treatment of carcinogenesis data, 119
  variation in incidence of spontaneous tumors, 3
susceptibility of different species, 42
Carcinogens,
  alkylating agents, 80
  chemotherapeutic agents, 96
  criteria, 55
  cytotoxicity, 91, 92
    dose–response relationship, 92
    lethality, 91
    morphological transformation, 92
    statistical analysis, 92
  definition, 41, 48
  direct-acting, 30
  effect on cellular homeostasis, 78
  emergency safety standards in industry, 10
  hepatic, 96
  hormonal, 47
  interaction with DNA, 86
  macromolecular binding, 86
  metabolism in human cell cultures, 115, 116
  metabolic activation, 75–78
  non-hepatic, 96
  positive controls, 29–34
    active intermediates, 30
    compounds in current use, 31–33
    consistency of response, 34
    correlation of negative results with sensitivity of test
      system, 30
    definition, 29
    disposal of residues, 30
    evaluation of relative sensitivities of bioassay systems,
      29, 30
    interpretation of indefinite response, 29
    number of test animals, 30
    potential hazards, 30

proximal, 46, 75, 77
  derivatives, 77
  effect of metabolic pathways, 75
  metabolism of test compound, 46
  reactions implicated, 77
regulation of use, 11
restrictions for use, 10
standard compounds used as positive controls, 34
tumorigenicity following prenatal exposure, 26
ultimate, 75, 77
  derivatives, 77
  effect of metabolic pathways, 75
  initiation of carcinogenesis, 75
  reactions implicated, 77
Carcinomas,
  adrenal cortical,
    incidence in inbred mouse strains, 60
  basal-cell, 6, 8
    incidence in CRCD control rats, 8
    spontaneous development in CRCD control rats, 6
  colonic,
    dietary effects mediated by intestinal flora, 19
  cutaneous, 6, 7, 51, 60, 61
    incidence in CRCD control rats, 7
    incidence in inbred mouse strains, 60, 61
    relation to drug exposure, 51
    spontaneous development in CRCD control rats, 6
  endometrial,
    relation to drug exposure, 51
  hepatic, undifferentiated,
    description, 72
  hepatocellular, 51, 71
    description, 71
    relation to drug exposure, 51
  islet-cell,
    spontaneous development in CRCD control rats, 6
  mammary, 19, 62, 73
    description, 73
    dietary effects mediated by intestinal flora, 19
    incidence in inbred mouse strains, 62
    incidence in wild mice, 62
  pituitary,
    incidence in CRCD control rats, 7
  prostatic,
    incidence in Sprague-Dawley and Fischer rats, 57
  renal, 6, 7, 64
    incidence in CRCD control rats, 7
    incidence in inbred mouse strains, 64
    spontaneous development in CRCD control rats, 6
  renal-cell,
    incidence in Sprague-Dawley and Fischer rats, 57
  renal-pelvis,
    relation to drug exposure, 51
  sebaceous-gland, 6, 7
    incidence in CRCD control rats, 7
    spontaneous development in CRCD control rats, 6
  sinal,
    relation to drug exposure, 51
  squamous-cell, 6–8, 57, 64
    incidence in CRCD control rats, 7, 8
    incidence in inbred mouse strains, 64
    incidence in Sprague-Dawley and Fischer rats, 57

    spontaneous development in CRCD control rats, 6
  thymic, 6, 7
    incidence in CRCD control rats, 7
    spontaneous development in CRCD control rats, 6
  transitional-cell, 6–8
    incidence in CRCD control rats, 7, 8
    spontaneous development in CRCD control rats, 6
  urocystic, 6–8, 51
    incidence in CRCD control rats, 7, 8
    relation to drug exposure, 51
    spontaneous development in CRCD control rats, 6
Cardiorespiratory tumors,
  incidence in Sprague-Dawley and Fischer rats, 58
Cartilaginous-tissue tumors,
  incidence in Sprague-Dawley and Fischer rats, 58
Casein level, dietary,
  correlation with protein and enzyme activity, 17
Cell cultures,
  alterations in mammalian cells, 91
  bioassay techniques, 109, 110
    epithelial cells, 109, 110
    hamster embryo system, 109
    limitations, 110
    mouse fibroblast cell lines, 109
    organ cultures, 110
  combined actions of chemicals with viruses or radiation,
    93
  host-mediated combination bioassay, 93
  in vitro carcinogenesis, 85, 86
    chemical transformation, 85
    malignant transformation, 85, 86
    morphological transformation, 85, 86
  materials of human origin, 115–117
    diploid embryonic lung, 115
    Down's syndrome, 115
    neurofibrosarcomas, 115
    whole embryo, 115
    xeroderma pigmentosum, 115
  metabolism of carcinogens in materials of human
    origin, 115, 116
  neoplastic transformations, 113, 114
  specific-locus mutational assay, 101
  transformation in Syrian hamster systems, 92
Cell-mediated immunity,
  effects of dietary deficiencies, 19
Cellular homeostasis,
  carcinogenic modification, 78
  effect of metabolic pathways, 75
Central nervous system,
  susceptibility of fetal tissue to carcinogens, 25
  tumor development following prenatal exposure to
    carcinogens, 23
Centrifugation analysis,
  measurement of DNA damage and repair, 97, 98
Cervical tumors,
  adenocarcinomas,
    relation to drug exposure, 51
  fibromas, 6
    incidence in CRCD control rats, 7
    spontaneous development in CRCD control rats, 6
Chemical-interaction measurements,
  animal models, 95

covalent binding, 95
crosslinks of DNA, 95
DNA damage,
  sedimentation analysis, 96
  unscheduled DNA repair synthesis, 96, 97
dominant-lethal test, 95
intercalation with DNA bases, 95
latent period, 95
microorganism test systems, 95
phosphate and amino groups of DNA, 95
strand breakage, 96
Chimpanzee,
  lymphoma-virus susceptibility, 67
Chinese hamster,
  somatic-cell assays, 104
Chloramphenicol,
  carcinogenic effects in man, 51, 53
  determination of mutagenicity, 85
  production of chromosomal defects, 53
Chlordane,
  inhibition of carcinogenesis, 19
Chlornaphazine,
  carcinogenic effect in man, 52
Chlorocarbons, 80
Cholangiocarcinomas,
  description, 72
Choline,
  effect on toxicity and carcinogenicity of chemicals, 17
Chondromas,
  incidence in Sprague-Dawley and Fischer rats, 58
Chow diets,
  effect on aryl hydrocarbon hydroxylase activity, 17
  inhibition of 2-AAF-induced tumors, 17
  nutrient variations, 18, 19
Chromosomal defects,
  production by chloramphenicol administration, 53
Chrysene,
  carcinogenic effect on cell cultures, 86
  relative carcinogenic activity, 39
  tumor-initiating activity, 37, 39
Cinnamon ringtail monkey,
  lymphoma-virus susceptibility, 67
Clitoral-gland tumors,
  incidence in inbred mouse strains, 64
CMI, see Cell-mediated immunity
Coal-tar preparations,
  carcinogenic effect in man, 51, 53
Cocarcinogens,
  effect on DNA repair, 76
Colchicine,
  carcinogenic activity, 81
Combination bioassay, host-mediated, 93
Compressed carcinogenicity tests,
  assay of enhanced tumor induction, 82
  initiation and promotion systems, 82
  transplacental carcinogenisis, 82, 83
Concretions, bladder, 42, 81
Contaminants, environmental,
  effect on tumor development in control animals, 56
Control animals,
  effect of environmental contaminants, 56
  spontaneous-tumor incidence, 2, 9

adrenal-gland pheochromocytomas, 9
  use of background data, 2
survey of spontaneous-tumor development, 5–9
variation of incidence of specific tumors, 9
Copper,
  content in chow diets, 18
Cortical tumors,
  adenomas, adrenal, 8, 57, 60
    incidence in CRCD control rats, 8
    incidence in inbred mouse strains, 60
    incidence in Sprague-Dawley and Fischer rats, 57
  adenomas, renal, 6, 7
    incidence in CRCD control rats, 7
    spontaneous development in CRCD control rats, 6
  carcinomas, adrenal,
    incidence in inbred mouse strains, 60
Corticosteroids,
  carcinogenic effect in man, 51, 52
Creosote preparations,
  carcinogenic effect in man, 53
Cricetulus griseus, see Chinese hamster
Croton oil,
  tumor promotion, 36
Cycasin,
  determination of mutagenicity, 85
  tumorigenicity following prenatal exposure, 25
Cyclophosphamide,
  carcinogenic effect in man, 52
Cystadenomas, mammary,
  incidence in CRCD control rats, 8
  spontaneous development in CRCD control rats, 6
Cytotoxic drugs,
  carcinogenic effects in man, 51, 52
  use in cancer chemotherapy, 52
Cytotoxicity,
  lethality, 91
  morphological transformation, 92
  statistical analysis, 92

D

DAB, see 4-Dimethylaminobenzene
DDT,
  content in chow diets, 18
Delaney clause, 11
N-Demethylase,
  correlation with dietary casein level, 17
Deoxyadenosine,
  covalent binding, 95
Deoxycytosine,
  covalent binding, 95
Deoxyguanosine,
  covalent binding, 95
Dermal tumors,
  incidence in Sprague-Dawley and Fischer rats, 57
Dibenz(a,h)anthracene,
  isolation from coal tar, 79
Dibutylnitrosamine,
  carcinogenic activity, 81
1,2-Diethylhydrazine,
  tumorigenicity following prenatal exposure, 26

Diethylnitrosamine,
  carcinogenic effect in rodents, 30
  induction of single-strand breaks in hepatic DNA, 96
  tumorigenicity following prenatal exposure, 26
  use as positive control compound, 30, 31
  use with murine leukemia virus, 86
Diethylstilbestrol,
  carcinogenicity following prenatal exposure, 23, 25
Diethylsulfate,
  tumorigenicity following prenatal exposure, 26
Diets,
  chow, 17, 18
    effect on aryl hydrocarbon hydroxylase activity, 17
    inhibition of 2-AAF-induced tumors, 17
    nutrient variations, 18
  correlation of casein level with protein and enzyme
      activity, 17
  fats, 17
  folate deficiency, 19
  folic acid deficiency, 19
  influence on spontaneous-tumor incidence, 55
  lipotrope deficiency, 17–19
    effect on aflatoxin B_1 toxicity and carcinogenicity,
      17, 18
    effect on cell-mediated immunity, 19
    effect on hepatic drug-metabolizing enzymes, 18
    effect on immunologic processes, 19
    effect on nitrosamine-induced carcinogenesis, 18
    effect on pyrorolizidine alkaloid toxicity, 17
  lipotropic nutrients, 17
  manipulation, 20
  mechanisms of action, 18, 19
  natural-product, 17
  protein deficiency, 17, 19
    effect on cell-mediated immunity, 19
    effect on immunologic processes, 19
    effect on tumor growth, 17, 19
    riboflavin deficiency, 17
    semisynthetic purified, 17
    standardization, 19, 20
    vitamin A deficiency, 18
Dilantin, see Diphenylhydantoin
Dimethylhydrazine,
  induction of DNA breaks, 96
4-Dimethylaminoazobenzene,
  enhancement of carcinogenesis by riboflavin deficiency,
    17
7,9-Dimethylbenz(c)acridine,
  carcinogenic activity, 81
Dimethylbenzanthracene,
  effect on nervous system in rats following prenatal
    exposure, 25
7,12-Dimethylbenz[a]anthracene,
  carcinogenic effect on cell cultures, 86
  inhibition of carcinogenicity, 19
  tumorigenicity following prenatal exposure, 26
  use as positive control compound, 32
  use with virus, 86
Dimethylhydrazine,
  effect of dietary vitamin A deficiency on carcino-
    genicity, 18
Dimethylnitrosamine,

carcinogenic activity, 82
carcinogenic effects in relation to timing of treatment,
    25
determination of mutagenicity, 85
induction of single-strand breaks in hepatic DNA, 96
tumorigenicity following prenatal exposure, 26
N,N-Dimethyl-4-stilbenamine,
  use as positive control compound, 32
Dimethylsulfate,
  tumorigenicity following prenatal exposure, 26
N,N-Dinitrosopiperazine,
  induction of single-strand breaks in hepatic DNA, 96
Diphenylhydantoin,
  carcinogenic effects in man, 51, 53
  concurrent depression and stimulation of immune
      response, 53
Diploid human cells,
  somatic-cell assays, 105
DMBA, see Dimethylbenzanthracene
DMN, see Dimethylnitrosamine
DNA damage,
  measurement, 96–99
    centrifugation analysis, 96, 97
    proposed method, 98, 99
    sedimentation analysis, 96
    unscheduled DNA repair synthesis, 96, 97
    unscheduled incorporation of radioactive precursors,
      96
  UV-induced, 84
DNA methylation, 86
DNA repair,
  assays for detection, 105, 106
  effect of 4-nitroquinoline-N-oxide, 87
  excision, 101, 102
    deficiency in Salmonella mutants, 102
    NCI prescreening study, 101
  inhibition, 76
  measurements, 98, 99, 105, 106
    ^{14}C-labeled-thymidine uptake into DNA, 105
    linkage of broken strands, 106
    proposed method, 98, 99
  synthesis, 96–99
    in hepatic cells, 96
    unscheduled, 96–98
    use as bioassay, 99
  UV-induced, 95
DNA target molecule,
  initiation of chemical carcinogenesis, 95
Dogs,
  distribution of spontaneous tumors with respect to
      anatomic sites, 65
  spontaneous tumor incidence, 65
Dosage levels,
  arbitrarily "safe" level, 43
  frequency, 22
  maximal tolerated dose, 47
  minimum effective dose, 42
  route of administration, 22
  selection, 21, 22
  "socially acceptable" level, 43
  test range for hormonal carcinogens, 47
  threshold dose, 42

WHO recommendations, 3, 4
Dose—response curves, 4
Dose—response relationship of cytotoxicity, 92
Drug effects, carcinogenic,
  design of experiments for detection, 1—12
  tissues affected by specific compounds, in man, 51—53
    arsenic, 51
    chloramphenicol, 51, 53
    coal-tar preparations, 51, 53
    cytotoxic drugs, 51, 52
    diphenylhydantoin, 51, 53
    hormones, 51, 52
    immunosuppressive drugs, 51, 52
    inorganic arsenicals, 52
    phenacetin-containing drugs, 51—53
    radioisotopes, 51
Duration of tests,
  inception, 23
  guidelines for establishment, 5
  neonatal treatment, 23
  prenatal exposure, 23, 25, 26
    carcinogenicity of diethylstilbestrol, 23, 25
    difference in target sites, 26
    integration with long-term postnatal exposure, 26
    metabolic competence of fetal tissue, 25
    nitrosamide-induced tumors, 23
    reduction in tumor-latency period, 26
    timing of treatment, 25
    tumorigenicity of nitrosamides, 23

E

Elasiomycin,
  tumorigenicity following prenatal exposure, 26
Endocrine tumors,
  incidence in Sprague-Dawley and Fischer rats, 57
Endometrial carcinomas,
  relation to drug exposure, 51
Environmental oncogens, 83
Epidemiologic studies, 41
Epithelial cell cultures,
  malignant and morphological transformations, 109, 110
Epoxides,
  association between carcinogenicity and mutagenicity, 104
Escherichia coli,
  in host-mediated assays, 84
  mutants, DNA polymerase-deficient, 102
Esophageal tumors,
  in hamsters, 29
Estrogens,
  carcinogenic effects, 83
Estrogens, synthetic,
  carcinogenic effects in man, 52
Ethylmethanesulfonate,
  induction of single-strand breaks in hepatic DNA, 96
Ethylnitrosobiuret,
  tumorigenicity following prenatal exposure, 26
Ethylnitrosourea,
  tumorigenicity following prenatal exposure, 26
N-Ethyl-N-nitrosourea,

induction of single-strand breaks in hepatic DNA, 96
Ethylnitrosourethane,
  tumorigenicity following prenatal exposure, 26
4-Ethylsulfonylnaphthalene-1-sulfonamide,
  carcinogenic activity, 81

F

Fat, dietary,
  effect on tumor growth, 17
Fibroadenomas,
  cutaneous, 6, 8
    incidence in CRCD control rats, 8
    spontaneous development in CRCD control rats, 6
  mammary, 6—8, 57
    incidence in CRCD control rats, 7, 8
    incidence in Sprague-Dawley and Fischer rats, 57
    spontaneous development in CRCD control rats, 6
Fibromas,
  cervical, 6, 7
    incidence in CRCD control rats, 7
    spontaneous development in CRCD control rats, 6
  dermal,
    incidence in Sprague-Dawley and Fischer rats, 57
  mammary,
    spontaneous development in CRCD control rats, 6
  periosteal,
    incidence in Sprague-Dawley and Fischer rats, 58
  striated-muscle,
    spontaneous development in CRCD control rats, 6
  various tissues,
    spontaneous development in CRCD control rats, 6
Fibrosarcomas,
  dermal,
    incidence in Sprague-Dawley and Fischer rats, 57
  skeletal-muscle,
    incidence in CRCD control rats, 9
  striated-muscle,
    spontaneous development in CRCD control rats, 6
  various tissues, 6, 7
    incidence in CRCD control rats, 7
    spontaneous development in CRCD control rats, 6
N-2-Fluorenylacetamide,
  carcinogenic effect in rodents, 30
  use as positive control compound, 30, 31
Folate deficiency, dietary,
  effect on cell-mediated immunity, 19
Folic acid,
  effect on toxicity and carcinogenicity of chemicals, 17
Folic acid deficiency, dietary,
  effect on immunologic processes, 19
Food additives,
  evaluation of safety, 45, 46
Food and Drug Administration,
  operating policy, 43, 46
    dose exaggeration, 46
    priorities in drug testing, 43
Formazan deposition test, 81
Forward mutation, determination of potency, 102
Frameshift mutations, detection, 102

G

Ganglioneuroblastomas, adrenal,
  incidence in Sprague-Dawley and Fischer rats, 57
Gastric tumors,
  leiomyosarcomas,
    incidence in Sprague-Dawley and Fischer rats, 58
  papillomas, 6, 7
    incidence in CRCD control rats, 7
    spontaneous development in CRCD control rats, 6
  various neoplasms,
    incidence in inbred mouse strains, 60
Genetic factors,
  sensitivity of carcinogenic response, 29
Gliomas, encephalic,
  incidence in CRCD control rats, 7, 8
  spontaneous development in CRCD control rats, 6
Gonadal dysgenesis,
  carcinogenic effect of treatment with stilbestrol, 52
Granular-cell myoblastomas,
  incidence in inbred mouse strains, 64
Granulocytic leukemia,
  incidence in inbred mouse strains, 63
Granulosa-cell tumors,
  incidence in CRCD control rats, 8
  incidence in inbred mouse strains, 62
  incidence in wild mice, 62
  spontaneous development in CRCD control rats, 6
Griseofulvin,
  carcinogenicity in test animals, 49
  effect on tumor development, 49
  interference with porphyrin metabolism, 42
  metabolic differences among animal species, 9, 10
Guanine utilization, 104

H

Hamster embryo system, 109
Hamsters,
  spontaneous-tumor incidence, 65
Harderian-gland tumors,
  incidence in inbred mouse strains, 60, 61, 63
Hemangioendotheliomas,
  hepatic, 51, 72
    description, 72
    relation to drug exposure, 51
  pulmonary,
    description, 72
  various tissues, 60, 61, 63
    incidence in inbred mouse strains, 60, 61, 63
    incidence in wild mice, 63
Hemangiosarcomas,
  incidence in CRCD control rats, 7
  spontaneous development in CRCD control rats, 6
Hematopoietic-system tumors,
  hemangiosarcomas, 6, 7
    incidence in CRCD control rats, 7
    spontaneous development in CRCD control rats, 6
  leukemia, 6, 51
    relation to drug exposure, 51
    spontaneous development in CRCD control rats, 6

Hemoproteins, CO-binding,
  association with enzyme activity, 76
Hepatic tumors,
  adenomas, 6, 7
    incidence in CRCD control rats, 7
    spontaneous development in CRCD control rats, 6
  cholangiocarcinomas,
    description, 72
  hemangioendotheliomas, 51, 72
    description, 72
    relation to drug exposure, 51
  hepatocellular adenomas,
    incidence in CRCD control rats, 8
  hepatocellular carcinomas, 51, 71
    description, 71
    relation to drug exposure, 51
  hepatomas, 49, 61, 62, 82
    assay in compressed carcinogenicity tests, 82
    effect of griseofulvin administration, 49
    incidence in inbred mouse strains, 61, 62
    incidence in wild mice, 62
  reticulum sarcomas,
    incidence in CRCD control rats, 8
  sarcomas,
    relation to drug exposure, 51
  undifferentiated carcinomas,
    description, 72
Hepatocarcinogens,
  DNA damage, 96
Hepatomas,
  assay in compressed carcinogenicity tests, 82
  effect of griseofulvin administration, 61
  incidence in inbred mouse strains, 59, 62
  incidence in wild mice, 62
Herpesviruses,
  effect of inoculation in monkeys, 66
  oncogenic range in monkeys, 67
Histidine locus, "hot spots", 102
Histiocytosis, malignant, 58
  incidence in Sprague-Dawley and Fischer rats, 58
HGPRT, see Hypoxanthine-guanine phosphoribosyl-
    transferase
Hodgkin's disease,
  carcinogenic effects of treatment, 52
Hormones,
  classification of chemical carcinogens, 80
  carcinogenic effects, 51, 52, 83
  influence on spontaneous-tumor incidence, 55
Host-mediated assay,
  method, 84, 85
  NCI prescreening study, 101
  results with *Salmonella typhimurium*, 85
Human cell-culture systems,
  culture conditions, 116, 117
  diploid embryonic lung, 115
  Down's syndrome, 115
  effect of benzo[a]pyrene, 116
  metabolism of carcinogens, 115, 116
  neurofibrosarcomas, 115
  selection of donor cells, 116
  whole embryo, 115
  xeroderma pigmentosum, 115

Hürthle-cell adenomas,
  incidence in Sprague-Dawley and Fischer rats, 57
Human lymphocyte lines,
  DNA repair, 106
  forward mutation, 105
Hycanthone,
  mutagenicity, 105
Hycanthone methanesulfonate,
  induction of single-strand breaks in hepatic DNA, 96
Hydrazides, 80
Hydrazine,
  carcinogenicity of derivatives, 48
  metabolic activity, 48
Hydrazine sulfate,
  effect on different mouse strains, 10
Hydrocarbons, polycyclic,
  association between carcinogenicity and mutagenicity,
    104
  carcinogenic effect in man, 53
  effect on cell cultures, 86
  inhibition of carcinogenesis, 19
  mutagenesis assessment, 102
  tumorigenicity following prenatal exposure, 25
Hydrocarbons, polycyclic aromatic,
  classification of chemical carcinogens, 80
  metabolism of methyl groups, 77
  oxide metabolism, 76
Hydrocarbons, polynuclear aromatic,
  content in combustion products, 35
  relative carcinogenic activity, 36–39
N-Hydroxy-2-acetylaminofluorene,
  induction of single-strand breaks in hepatic DNA, 96
4-Hydroxyaminoquinoline-N-oxide,
  induction of single-strand breaks in hepatic DNA, 96
N-Hydroxy-N-2-fluorenylacetamide,
  effect of administration on hamsters, 29
Hydroxylamine,
  determination of mutagenicity, 85
3-Hydroxyxanthine,
  induction of single-strand breaks in hepatic DNA, 96
Hyperplasia, urocystic epithelium, 81, 82
Hyperplasia test, 81
Hypoxanthine-guanine phosphoribosyl transferase,
  deficiency in mutant hamster cells, 104
Hypoxanthine utilization, 104

I

Iatrogenic cancer,
  potential hazards of therapeutic drugs, 49
Immune response,
  concurrent depression and stimulation by diphenyl-
    hydantoin, 53
Immunologic factors,
  influence on development of induced tumors, 55, 56
  influence on spontaneous-tumor incidence, 55, 56
Immunologic processes,
  relationship to dietary effects on carcinogenesis, 19
Immunologic surveillance,
  inhibition by immunosuppressive drugs, 51
Immunostimulation,

interaction with immunosuppression, 52
Immunosuppressive drugs,
  carcinogenic effect in man, 51, 52
  interaction with immunostimulation, 52
Induction of neoplasia,
  alteration of mammalian cells in culture, 91
  combined action of chemicals with viruses or radiation,
    92, 93
  cross-band pattern of chromosomes, 92
  end point of cell cultures, 91
  false negatives and false positives, 92, 93
  host-mediated combination bioassay, 93
  lethality of cells, 91, 92
  morphological transformation, 92
  predictability of tumor production, 91
  quantitation of transformed cell, 91
  statistical analysis of transformation frequency, 92
Informational target molecules,
  interaction with carcinogenic agents, 78
INH, see Isoniazid
Inorganics, 80
Interstitial-cell tumors,
  incidence in CRCD control rats, 8
  incidence in inbred mouse strains, 60
  incidence in Sprague-Dawley and Fischer rats, 57
  spontaneous development in CRCD control rats, 6
Intestinal flora,
  relationship to dietary effects on carcinogenesis, 19
In vitro tests,
  host-mediated assay, 84, 85
  macromolecular binding of carcinogens and DNA
    repair, 86, 87
  phases of chemical carcinogenesis, 83
  transformation of cell cultures, 85, 86
  tumor progression, 87
In vivo tests,
  compressed carcinogenicity tests, 82, 83
  formazan deposition test, 81
  hyperplasia test, 81
  sebaceous-gland suppression test, 81
  subacute toxicity tests, 81, 82
Iodine,
  content in chow diets, 18
Irradiation,
  pathogenesis of tumorigenic effect, 42
Islet-cell tumors,
  incidence in CRCD control rats, 8
  incidence in inbred mouse strains, 64
  incidence in Sprague-Dawley and Fischer rats, 57
Isoniazid, 48
N-Isopropyl-α-(2-methylhydrazine)-p-toluamide,
  tumorigenicity following prenatal exposure, 26

K

Keratoacanthomas,
  incidence in CRCD control rats, 7, 8
  spontaneous development in CRCD control rats, 6
Kidney transplants,
  carcinogenic effects of immunosuppressive drugs, 51,
    52

Kidney tumors,
  adenomas,
    incidence in CRCD control rats, 8
  carcinomas, 6, 7, 64
    incidence in CRCD control rats, 7
    incidence in inbred mouse strains, 64
    spontaneous development in CRCD control rats, 6
  cortical adenomas, 6, 7
    incidence in CRCD control rats, 7
    spontaneous development in CRCD control rats, 6

L

Latent period,
  dose-dependence, 11
  proportion of total life span, 11
  reduction in prenatal exposure, 26
Leaky allele, 103
Leiomyomas,
  dermal,
    incidence in Sprague-Dawley and Fischer rats, 57
  uterine, 57, 63
    incidence in inbred mouse strains, 63
    incidence in Sprague-Dawley and Fischer rats, 57
Leiomyosarcomas,
  dermal,
    incidence in Sprague-Dawley and Fischer rats, 57
  gastric,
    incidence in Sprague-Dawley and Fischer rats, 58
  vaginal, 6, 7
    incidence in control rats, 7
    spontaneous development in CRCD control rats, 6
Lesch-Nyhan syndrome, 105
Leukemia,
  classification, 72
  description, 72, 73
  incidence in CRCD control rats, 9
  incidence in inbred mouse strains, 59, 61, 63
  incidence in Sprague-Dawley and Fischer rats, 58
  relation to drug exposure, 51
  spontaneous development in CRCD control rats, 6
Leukemogenic agents,
  potential to produce aplastic anemia, 53
Light-cell tumors, thyroid,
  incidence in Sprague-Dawley and Fischer rats, 57
Lipomas,
  cutaneous,
    incidence in CRCD control rats, 8
  various tissues,
    spontaneous development in CRCD control rats, 6
Liposarcomas,
  incidence in CRCD control rats, 7
  spontaneous development in CRCD control rats, 6
Lipotrope deficiency, dietary,
  effect in aflatoxin B_1 toxicity and carcinogenicity, 17, 18
  effect on cell-mediated immunity, 19
  effect on hepatic drug-metabolizing enzymes, 18
  effect on immunologic processes, 19
  effect on nitrosamine-induced carcinogenesis, 18
  effect on pyrorolizidine alkaloid toxicity, 17

Lung cancer,
  excessive use of tobacco, 29
Lung tumors,
  adenocarcinomas,
    description, 72
  adenomas, 48, 72, 82
    assay in compressed carcinogenicity tests, 82
    description, 72
    effect of isoniazid administration, 48
    effect of metronidazole administration, 48
    induction by 1-acetyl-1-isonicotinoylhydrazine in mice, 48
  hemangioendothelial sarcomas,
    description, 72
  lymphosarcomas, 6, 7
    incidence in CRCD control rats, 7
    spontaneous development in CRCD control rats, 6
  non-chromaffin paragangliomas, 6, 8
    incidence in CRCD control rats, 8
    spontaneous development in CRCD control rats, 6
  primary, 59, 61, 62
    incidence in inbred mouse strains, 59, 61, 62
    incidence in wild mice, 62
Luteomas,
  incidence in inbred mouse strains, 62
Lymphocytic leukemia,
  incidence in inbred mouse strains, 61
Lymphocytic neoplasms,
  incidence in inbred mouse strains, 63
  incidence in wild mice, 63
Lymphomas,
  splenic, 6, 8
    incidence in CRCD control rats, 8
    spontaneous development in CRCD control rats, 6
  spontaneous,
    occurrence and etiology in monkeys, 66
  various tissues, 6, 7, 15, 48, 51, 72
    classification, 72
    description, 72
    effect of isoniazid administration, 48
    effect of metronidazole administration, 48
    incidence in CRCD control rats, 7
    recommended test strain, mouse, 15
    relation to drug exposure, 51
    spontaneous development in CRCD control rats, 6
Lymphoma viruses,
  effect of inoculation in monkeys, 66
  oncogenic range in monkeys, 67
Lymphoreticular tumors,
  incidence in Sprague-Dawley and Fischer rats, 58
Lymphosarcomas,
  pulmonary, 6, 7
    incidence in CRCD control rats, 7
    spontaneous development in CRCD control rats, 6
  various tissues,
    spontaneous development in CRCD control rats, 6

M

Malignancy,
  criteria, 71

differentiation, 71
hepatic tumors, 71, 72
leukemias, 72, 73
lymphomas, 72
mammary-gland tumors, 73
pulmonary tumors, 72
Malignant neurofibrosarcomas,
  spontaneous conversion from benign neurofibromas,
    115
Malignant transformation, definition, 85, 109
Malignant tumors, definition, 41
Marmosets,
  lymphoma-virus susceptibility, 67
Mast-cell neoplasms,
  incidence in wild mice, 63
Mammalian assay systems, 101
Mammalian culture systems,
  bioassay techniques, 109, 110
    epithelial fibroblast cells, 109, 110
    hamster embryo system, 109
    mouse fibroblast cell lines, 109
    organ cultures, 110
  DNA repair, 105, 106
  somatic-cell assay, 104, 105
    Chinese hamster, 104
    diploid human cells, 105
    human lymphoblastoid cells, 105
    mouse lymphoma cells, 104, 105
Mammary-gland tumors,
  adenocanthomas,
    incidence in inbred mice, 62
  adenocarcinomas, 6–9, 57
    differences in incidence between control groups of
      CRCD rats, 9
    incidence in CRCD control rats, 7, 8
    incidence in Sprague-Dawley and Fischer rats, 57
    spontaneous development in CRCD control rats, 6
  adenomas, 6–8, 57
    incidence in CRCD control rats, 7, 8
    incidence in Sprague-Dawley and Fischer rats, 57
    spontaneous development in CRCD control rats, 6
  carcinomas, 62, 73
    description, 73
    incidence in inbred mouse strains, 62
    incidence in wild mice, 62
  cystadenomas, 6, 8
    incidence in CRCD control rats, 8
    spontaneous development in CRCD control rats, 6
  fibroadenomas, 6–8, 57
    incidence in CRCD control rats, 7, 8
    incidence in Sprague-Dawley and Fischer rats, 57
    spontaneous development in CRCD control rats, 6
  fibromas,
    spontaneous development in CRCD control rats, 6
  neoplasms,
    incidence in inbred mouse strains, 59
  papillary cystadenocarcinomas, 6, 8
    incidence in CRCD control rats, 8
    spontaneous development in CRCD control rats, 6
  papillary cystadenomas, 6, 8
    incidence in CRCD control rats, 8
    spontaneous development in CRCD control rats, 6

sarcomas,
  incidence in inbred mouse strains, 64
various types,
  incidence in inbred mouse strains, 61
Maximal tolerated dose, 47
Melphalan,
  carcinogenic effect in man, 52
Mesotheliomas, abdominal,
  incidence in Sprague-Dawley and Fischer rats, 58
Mesothorium,
  carcinogenic effect in man, 51
Metabolic activation,
  in carcinogenic response, 75–78
    balance between pathways, 76
    CO-binding hemoproteins, 76
    interaction with targets, 75
    manipulation of pathways, 78
    reactivity with cellular macromolecules, 78
  relation to species, strain, and dietary influences in
    carcinogenesis, 83
Metals, 80
Methionine,
  effect on toxicity and carcinogenicity of chemicals, 17
Methylation of DNA, 86
Methylaxozymethanol acetate,
  induction of single-strand breaks in hepatic DNA, 96
  induction of DNA breaks, 96
  tumorigenicity following prenatal exposure, 26
3-Methylbenz[a]anthracene,
  carcinogenic effect on cell cultures, 86
8-Methylbenz[a]anthracene,
  carcinogenic effect on cell cultures, 86
10-Methylbenz[a]anthracene,
  carcinogenic effect on cell cultures, 86
1-Methyl-2-benzylhydrazine,
  tumorigenicity following prenatal exposure, 26
Methylcholanthrene,
  tumorigenicity following prenatal exposure, 26
3-Methylcholanthrene,
  effect on cell cultures, 85, 86
  use with virus, 86
Methylchrysenes,
  carcinogenic activity, 38
  tumor-initiating activity, 37
3'-Methyl-4-dimethylaminoazobenzene,
  DNA repair synthesis in hepatic cells, 96
  induction of single-strand breaks in hepatic DNA, 96
  inhibition of carcinogenicity, 19
  use as positive control compound, 32
Methylmethanesulfonate,
  induction of single-strand breaks in hepatic DNA, 96
  tumorigenicity following prenatal exposure, 26
N'-Methyl-N'-nitro-N-nitrosoguanidine,
  determination of mutagenicity, 85
  levels of DNA repair synthesis in xeroderma pigmento-
    sum, 87
  use as positive control compound, 30
N-Methyl-N-nitroso-N'-nitroguanidine,
  induction of single-strand breaks in hepatic DNA, 96
N-Methyl-N-nitrosourea,
  induction of single-strand breaks in hepatic DNA, 96
Methylnitrosourethane,

induction of single-strand breaks in hepatic DNA, 96
Methyltestosterone,
  carcinogenic effect in man, 52
Metronidazole, 48
Mitomycin C,
  determination of mutagenicity, 85
Mouse fibroblast cell lines, 109
Mouse lymphoma,
  somatic-cell assays, 104, 105
Mouse strains,
  129,
    incidence of testicular teratomas, 60, 61
  A, 15, 59–61, 82
    assay of pulmonary adenomas, 82
    incidence of interstitial-cell tumors, 60
    incidence of mammary-gland tumors, 59, 61
    incidence of myoepitheliomas, 60, 61
    incidence of lung tumors, 59, 61
    tumor specificity, 15
  AKR,
    incidence of leukemia, 59, 61
  BALB/3T3,
    transformation of cell cultures, 92
  BALB/c, 15, 59–61
    incidence of hemangioendotheliomas, 60
    incidence of interstitial-cell tumors, 60
    incidence of mammary-gland tumors, 59
    incidence of myoepitheliomas, 60, 61
    incidence of lung tumors, 59
    tumor specificity, 15
  BL,
    incidence of lung tumors, 59
  BRS,
    incidence of stomach lesions, 60
  BRSUNT,
    incidence of stomach lesions, 60
  C3H, 15, 48, 59–61, 82, 86
    assay of hepatomas, 82
    incidence of Harderian-gland tumors, 60, 61
    incidence of hepatomas, 59
    incidence of mammary-gland tumors, 59, 61
    incidence of subcutaneous sarcomas, 60
    inhibition of mammary-gland tumors by isoniazid,
      48
    prostatic tissue in culture treatment, 86
    tumor specificity, 15
  C3H/J,
    incidence of subcutaneous sarcomas, 61
  C3He, 59, 60
    incidence of hepatomas, 59
    incidence of ovarian tumors, 60
  C3HeB,
    incidence of hepatomas, 61
  C3HeB/De, 61–64
    incidence of adenocanthomas, 62
    incidence of adrenal cortical tumors, 63
    incidence of Harderian-gland tumors, 63
    incidence of hemangioendotheliomas, 63
    incidence of hepatomas, 62
    incidence of lymphocytic neoplasms, 63
    incidence of mammary carcinomas, 62
    incidence of myoepitheliomas, 64

  incidence of ovarian tumors, 61, 62
  incidence of pheochromocytomas, 63
  incidence of plasma-cell neoplasms, 63
  incidence of primary lung tumors, 62
  incidence of reticulum-cell neoplasms, 62
  incidence of skin tumors, 64
  incidence of subcutaneous sarcomas, 63
  incidence of uterine tumors, 63
  C3HeB/Fe,
    incidence of ovarian tumors, 61
  C3Hf,
    incidence of hepatomas, 59
  C3Hf/He, 62–64
    incidence of adenocanthomas, 62
    incidence of granular myoblastomas, 64
    incidence of hemangioendotheliomas, 63
    incidence of hepatomas, 62
    incidence of lymphocytic neoplasms, 63
    incidence of mammary carcinomas, 62
    incidence of osteogenic sarcomas, 63
    incidence of ovarian tumors, 62
    incidence of primary lung tumors, 62
    incidence of renal carcinomas, 64
    incidence of reticulum-cell neoplasms, 62
    incidence of skin tumors, 64
    incidence of subcutaneous sarcomas, 63
    incidence of urocystic papillomas, 64
    incidence of uterine tumors, 63
  C57Bk,
    tumor specificity, 15
  C57BL, 60, 61
    incidence of pituitary adenomas, 60
    incidence of reticulum-cell neoplasms, 61
  C57BL/He, 62–64
    incidence of clitoral-gland tumors, 64
    incidence of hemangioendotheliomas, 63
    incidence of hepatomas, 62
    incidence of lymphocytic neoplasms, 63
    incidence of mammary carcinomas, 62
    incidence of ovarian tumors, 62
    incidence of primary lung tumors, 62
    incidence of reticulum-cell neoplasms, 62
    incidence of skin tumors, 64
    incidence of uterine tumors, 63
  C57BR/ed,
    incidence of pituitary-gland tumors, 61
  C57L, 59, 61
    incidence of pituitary-gland tumors, 61
    incidence of reticular-cell neoplasms, 59
  C57xC3H,
    tumor specificity, 15
  C58,
    incidence of leukemia, 59, 61
  CBA,
    incidence of subcutaneous sarcomas, 60
  CC57BR,
    incidence of mammary-gland tumors, 59
  CC57W,
    incidence of mammary-gland tumors, 59
  CE, 60, 61
    incidence of adrenal cortical tumors, 60, 61
    incidence of ovarian tumors, 61

CxA,
  tumor specificity, 15
DBA,
  incidence of mammary-gland tumors, 59
DBA/2,
  incidence of mammary-gland tumors, 61
DBA/2cBDe, 62, 63
  incidence of adrenal cortical tumors, 63
  incidence of granulocytic leukemia, 63
  incidence of Harderian-gland tumors, 63
  incidence of hemangioendotheliomas, 63
  incidence of hepatomas, 62
  incidence of lymphocytic neoplasms, 63
  incidence of mammary carcinomas, 62
  incidence of plasma-cell neoplasms, 63
  incidence of primary lung tumors, 62
  incidence of reticulum-cell neoplasms, 62
  incidence of subcutaneous sarcomas, 63
  incidence of uterine tumors, 63
DD,
  incidence of mammary-gland tumors, 61
F_1 hybrids,
  tumor specificity, 15
HE/De,
  incidence of skin carcinomas, 61
HR,
  incidence of hemangioendotheliomas, 60
  incidence of skin papillomas, 60
HR/De, 61–64
  incidence of Harderian-gland tumors, 63
  incidence of hemangioendotheliomas, 61, 63
  incidence of hepatomas, 62
  incidence of islet-cell tumors, 64
  incidence of lymphocytic neoplasms, 63
  incidence of mammary-gland tumors, 62, 64
  incidence of myoepitheliomas, 64
  incidence of ovarian tumors, 62
  incidence of primary lung tumors, 62
  incidence of reticulum-cell neoplasms, 62
  incidence of skin tumors, 61, 64
  incidence of teratomas, 64
  incidence of uterine tumors, 63
I,
  incidence of skin tumors, 60
  incidence of stomach lesions, 60
NH,
  incidence of adrenal cortical tumors, 60
RHI, 59, 61
  incidence of mammary-gland tumors, 59
  incidence of ovarian tumors, 61
SJL,
  incidence of reticulum-cell neoplasms, 61
SWR,
  incidence of lung tumors, 59, 61
wild, 62–64
  incidence of hemangioendotheliomas, 63
  incidence of hepatomas, 62
  incidence of lymphocytic neoplasms, 63
  incidence of mammary carcinomas, 62
  incidence of mast-cell neoplasms, 63
  incidence of osteogenic sarcomas, 63
  incidence of ovarian tumors, 62

incidence of pheochromocytomas, 63
incidence of primary lung tumors, 62
incidence of reticulum-cell neoplasms, 62
incidence of subcutaneous sarcomas, 63
incidence of teratomas, 64
Multiple myeloma,
  carcenogenic effects of treatment with cytotoxic drugs,
    52
Mutagenesis assessment,
  forward mutation, 102–105
    APRT locus, 105
    determination of potency, 102, 103
    effect of physical mutagens, 104
    enzyme involvement, 104
    induction in mouse lymphoma cells, 105
    occurrence in diploid human cells, 105
  genetic alteration, 102
  HGPRT deficiency in diploid human cells, 105
  proposed assay systems, 101
  resistance to 8-azaguanine in diploid human cells, 105
  reverse mutations, 102, 104
    determination of potency, 102
    effect of physical mutagens, 104
    enzyme involvement, 104
  testing of metabolites, 101
Mutagenic tests,
  lack of correlation for determining carcinogenic poten-
    tial, 1
  relation between carcinogenesis and mutation, 84
Myoblastoma, granular,
  incidence in inbred mouse strains, 64
Myoepitheliomas,
  incidence in inbred mouse strains, 60, 61, 64
Myelogenous leukemia,
  incidence in CRCD control rats, 9
Myelomonocytic leukemia, acute,
  relation to drug exposure, 51

N

β-Naphthoflavone,
  inhibition of carcinogenesis, 19
β-Naphthylamine,
  carcinogenic effect in man, 52
  susceptibility of different species, 42
Natulan, *see* Procarbazine
Natural-product diets,
  inhibition of 2-AAF-induced tumors, 17
Neocarzinostatin,
  determination of mutagenicity, 85
Neoplastic transformation,
  criteria in vitro, 113, 114
    agglutination by plant lectins, 114
    antigenic alterations, 114
    cloning efficiency, 114
    growth of transformed cells in soft agar, 113
    immortality of transformed cells, 113
    karyotypic changes, 114
    loss of contact inhibition, 114
    morphologic and growth characteristics, 113, 114
    production of biologically malignant neoplasms, 113

criteria in vivo, 113
Neural tumors,
   incidence in Sprague-Dawley and Fischer rats, 57
Neurofibromas,
   incidence in Sprague-Dawley and Fischer rats, 57
Neurofibrosarcomas,
   incidence in CRCD control rats, 7
   spontaneous development in CRCD control rats, 6
Neurospora,
   in host-mediated assays, 84
Neurospora crassa,
   ad-3 mutations, 103
New Zealand white rabbit,
   lymphoma-virus susceptibility, 67
Nitrates,
   content in chow diets, 18
Nitrogen mustard,
   use as positive control compound, 32
4-Nitroquinoline-N-oxide,
   induction of single-strand breaks in hepatic DNA, 96
   levels of DNA repair synthesis in xeroderma pigmento-
      sum, 87
4-Nitroquinoline-N-oxide derivatives,
   correlation between carcinogenicity and thymidine
      uptake, 106
Nitrosamides,
   effect of prenatal exposure, 23
Nitrosamine,
   effect of dietary lipotrope deficiency on carcinogenesis,
      18
Nitroso compounds,
   association between carcinogenicity and mutagenicity,
      104
N-Nitroso compounds,
   classification of chemical carcinogens, 80
   tumorigenicity following prenatal exposure, 25
Nitrosodihydrosouracil,
   induction of single-strand breaks in hepatic DNA, 96
Nitrosomethylurea,
   tumorigenicity following prenatal exposure, 26
Nitrosomethylurethane,
   tumorigenicity following prenatal exposure, 26
N-Nitrosomorpholine,
   induction of single-strand breaks in hepatic DNA, 96
N-Nitrosopiperidine,
   induction of single-strand breaks in hepatic DNA, 96
"No effect" level, 11
Non-chromaffin paragangliomas,
   incidence in CRCD control rats, 8
   spontaneous development in CRCD control rats, 6
Non-leaky allele, 103

O

Odontomas,
   incidence in CRCD control rats, 7
   spontaneous development in CRCD control rats, 6
Organ cultures,
   criteria for transformation, 110
   limitations, 110
   materials of human origin, 117

Osteogenic sarcomas,
   incidence in CRCD control rats, 7, 9
   incidence in inbred mouse strains, 63
   incidence in wild mice, 63
   relation to drug exposure, 51
   spontaneous development in CRCD control rats, 6
Ovarian tumors,
   adenomas, tubular,
      incidence in inbred mouse strains, 62
   arrhenoblastomas,
      incidence in Sprague-Dawley and Fischer rats, 57
   granulosa-cell tumors, 6, 8, 62
      incidence in CRCD control rats, 8
      incidence in inbred mouse strains, 62
      incidence in wild mice, 62
      spontaneous development in CRCD control rats, 6
   luteomas,
      incidence in inbred mouse strains, 62
   papillary cystadenocarcinomas, 6, 8, 62
      incidence in CRCD control rats, 8
      incidence in inbred mouse strains, 62
      spontaneous development in CRCD control rats, 6
   various types,
      incidence in inbred mouse strains, 60, 61
Owl monkey,
   lymphoma-virus susceptibility, 67
Oxymetholone,
   carcinogenic effect in man, 52

P

PAH, *see* Polynuclear aromatic hydrocarbons
Pancreatic tumors,
   acinar-cell adenomas, 6, 8
      incidence in CRCD control rats, 8
      spontaneous development in CRCD control rats, 6
   adenomas,
      spontaneous development in CRCD control rats, 6
   adenosarcomas,
      incidence in CRCD control rats, 7
   islet-cell, 6–8, 57
      incidence in CRCD control rats, 7, 8
      incidence in inbred mouse strains, 64
      incidence in Sprague-Dawley and Fischer rats, 57
      spontaneous development in CRCD control rats, 6
Papillary cystadenocarcinomas,
   mammary, 6, 8
      incidence in CRCD control rats, 8
      spontaneous development in CRCD control rats, 6
   ovarian, 6, 8
      incidence in CRCD control rats, 8
      spontaneous development in CRCD control rats, 6
Papillary cystadenomas,
   mammary, 6, 8
      incidence in CRCD control rats, 8
      spontaneous development in CRCD control rats, 6
   ovarian,
      incidence in inbred mouse strains, 62
Papillomas,
   cutaneous, 6, 7, 60, 61, 64
      incidence in CRCD control rats, 7

incidence in inbred mouse strains, 60, 61, 64
spontaneous development in CRCD control rats, 6
gastric, 6, 7
incidence in CRCD control rats, 7
spontaneous development in CRCD control rats, 6
renal-pelvis,
incidence in Sprague-Dawley and Fischer rats, 57
urocystic, 57, 64
incidence in inbred mouse strains, 64
incidence in Sprague-Dawley and Fischer rats, 57
Parathyroid tumors,
spontaneous development in CRCD control rats, 6
Particulates of respiratory pollutants, 35
Pathology procedures in carcinogenic studies, 5
Periosteal fibromas,
incidence in Sprague-Dawley and Fischer rats, 58
Peripheral nervous system,
tumor development following prenatal exposure to
carcinogens, 23
Phenacetin-containing drugs,
carcinogenic effects in man, 51−53
Phenobarbital,
inhibition of carcinogenesis, 19
increased microsomal enzyme activity, 19
1-Phenyl-3,3-diethyltriazene,
tumorigenicity following prenatal exposure, 26
1-Phenyl-3,3-dimethyltriazine,
tumorigenicity following prenatal exposure, 26
Pheochromocytomas,
difference in incidence between control groups of
CRCD rats, 9
incidence in CRCD control rats, 7, 8
incidence in inbred mouse strains, 63
incidence in Sprague-Dawley and Fischer rats, 57
incidence in wild mice, 63
spontaneous development in CRCD control rats, 6
^{32}P-Phosphate,
tumorigenicity following prenatal exposure, 26
Phosphorus, radioactive,
carcinogenic effect in man, 51
Pituitary-gland tumors,
adenocarcinomas, 6, 8
incidence in CRCD control rats, 8
spontaneous development in CRCD control rats, 6
adenomas, 6−9, 57, 60
differences in incidence between control groups of
CRCD rats, 9
incidence in CRCD control rats, 7, 8
incidence in inbred mouse strains, 60
incidence in Sprague-Dawley and Fischer rats, 57
spontaneous development in CRCD control rats, 6
carcinomas,
incidence in CRCD control rats, 7
various types,
incidence in inbred mouse strains, 61
Plasma-cell neoplasms,
incidence in inbred mouse strains, 63
Polycyclic hydrocarbons,
association between carcinogenicity and mutagenicity,
104
carcinogenic effect in man, 53
effect on cell cultures, 86

inhibition of carcinogenesis, 19
mutagenesis assessment, 102
tumorigenicity following prenatal exposure, 25
Polycyclic hydrocarbons, aromatic,
classification of chemical carcinogens, 80
metabolism of methyl groups, 77
oxide metabolism, 76
Polycythemia vera,
carcinogenic effects of treatment, 51, 52
with cytotoxic agents, 52
with radioisotopes, 51
Polynuclear aromatic hydrocarbons,
content in combustion products, 35
relative carcinogenic activity, 36−39
Polyps, uterine,
incidence in CRCD control rats, 7, 8
spontaneous development in CRCD control rats, 6
Positive controls,
active intermediates, 30
application, 10
compounds in current use, 31−33
consistency of response, 34
correlation of negative results with sensitivity of test
system, 30
definition, 29
evaluation of relative sensitivities of bioassay systems,
29, 30
in environmental respiratory carcinogenesis, 35−39
interpretation of indefinite response, 29
laboratory hazards, 10, 30
disposal of residues, 30
restrictions for use of carcinogens, 10
number of test animals, 30
stated purpose, 10
use of historical background data, 10
Precarcinogens, 97
Predictability of tumor production, 91
Prescreening tests,
mutagenesis assessment, 101−106
National Cancer Institute study, 101
procedural characteristics, 101
Primates,
use for bioassays, 15
Procarbazine,
tumorigenicity following prenatal exposure, 26
Promoting agents,
correlation between potency and carcinogenic activity,
110
1,3-Propane sulfone,
tumorigenicity following prenatal exposure, 26
β-Propiolactone,
carcinogenic activity, 81
n-Propylnitrosourea,
tumorigenicity following prenatal exposure, 26
Prostatic tumors,
carcinogenic effect of treatment with stilbestrol, 52
incidence in Sprague-Dawley and Fischer rats, 57
Protein,
correlation with dietary casein level, 17
Protein deficiency, dietary,
effect on immunologic processes, 19
effect on tumor growth, 17

Purines, 104
Pyrene,
  carcinogenic effect on cell cultures, 86
1-Pyridyl-3,3-diethyltriazene,
  tumorigenicity following prenatal exposure, 26
Pyrimidines, 104
Pyrrolizidine alkaloids,
  inhibition of acute toxicity by dietary lipotrope
     deficiency, 17

Q

Quantitation of transformed cells, 91

R

Radiation,
  combined action with chemicals, 93
  potential to produce aplastic anemia, 53
Radiation effects, 84
Radiochemicals, 80
Radioisotopes, 51
Radiomimetic drugs,
  pathogenesis of tumorigenic effect, 42
Radium, 51
Rat strains,
  BD, 123
  AXC, 15
  Fischer, 57, 58
    characteristic spontaneous tumors, 57, 58
  Sprague-Dawley, 57, 58
    characteristic spontaneous tumors, 57, 58
Renal-cell carcinomas,
  incidence in Sprague-Dawley and Fischer rats, 57
Renal-pelvis tumors,
  incidence in Sprague-Dawley and Fischer rats, 57
  relation to drug exposure in man, 51
Respiratory pollutants, 35
Reticulum-cell tumors,
  incidence in CRCD control rats, 8
  incidence in inbred mouse strains, 59, 61, 62
  incidence in wild mice, 62
  incidence in Sprague-Dawley and Fischer rats, 58
  relation to drug exposure, 51
  spontaneous development in CRCD control rats, 8
Reverse mutation, 102
Rhabdomyosarcomas,
  incidence in Sprague-Dawley and Fischer rats, 58
Rhesus monkey,
  lymphoma-virus susceptibility, 67
Riboflavin,
  content in chow diets, 18
Riboflavin deficiency, dietary,
  effect on DAB carcinogenesis, 17
Rosenkranz test, 102

S

Saccharomyces cerevisiae,
  mitotic recombinations, 103

  use as positive control compound, 30, 33
Safrole, 30, 33
Salivary-gland tumors,
  incidence in CRCD control rats, 7
  spontaneous development in CRCD control rats, 6
Salmonella,
  histidine-requiring mutants, 102, 103
Salmonella typhimurium,
  in host-mediated assays, 84, 85
Sarcomas,
  cutaneous,
    relation to drug exposure, 51
  endometrial,
    incidence in inbred mouse strains, 63
  hepatic,
    relation to drug exposure, 51
  hepatic, hemangioendothelial,
    description, 72
  hepatic reticular,
    incidence in CRCD control rats, 8
  histiocytic,
    incidence in Sprague-Dawley and Fischer rats, 58
  mammary,
    incidence in inbred mouse strains, 64
  osteogenic, 6, 7, 9, 63
    incidence in CRCD control rats, 7, 9
    incidence in inbred mouse strains, 63
    incidence in wild mice, 63
    spontaneous development in CRCD control rats, 6
  reticulum-cell, 6, 8; 58
    incidence in CRCD control rats, 8
    incidence in Sprague-Dawley and Fischer rats, 58
    spontaneous development in CRCD control rats, 6
  soft-tissue,
    relation to drug exposure, 51
  subcutaneous,
    incidence in inbred mouse strains, 60, 61, 63
    incidence in wild mice, 63
  thymic, 6, 7
    incidence in CRCD control rats, 7
    spontaneous development in CRCD control rats, 6
  uterine, 6, 7
    incidence in CRCD control rats, 7
    spontaneous development in CRCD control rats, 6
  various tissues, 6, 7
    incidence in CRCD control rats, 7
    spontaneous development in CRCD control rats, 6
Scrotal skin cancer, 91
Sebaceous-gland suppression test, 81
Sebaceous-gland tumors,
  incidence in CRCD control rats, 7
  spontaneous development in CRCD control rats, 6
Sedimentation analysis, 96
Semisynthetic diets, purified,
  formulation and use, 19, 20
  tumor yield, 17
Short-term tests,
  assessment of DNA damage and repair synthesis, 124
  cell cultures, 124
  chemical-interaction measurements, 95–99
    sedimentation analysis, 96–98
    unscheduled DNA synthesis, 96–99

criteria, 79, 80
induction of neoplasia, 91–93
  combined action of chemicals with viruses or radia-
    tion, 92, 93
  alteration of mammalian cells, 91
  cross-band pattern of chromosomes, 92
  end point of cell cultures, 91
  false negatives, 92, 93
  false positives, 92, 93
  host-mediated combination bioassay, 93
  lethality of cells, 91, 92
  morphological transformation, 92
  predictability of tumor production, 91
  quantitation of transformed cells, 91
  statistical analysis of transformation frequency, 92
in vitro tests, 82–87
  host-mediated assay, 84, 85
  macromolecular binding of carcinogens and DNA
    repair, 86, 87
  phases of chemical carcinogenesis, 83
  transformation of cell cultures, 85, 86
  tumor progression, 87
in vivo tests, 80–83
  compressed carcinogenicity tests, 82, 83
  formazan deposition test, 81
  hyperplasia tests, 81
  sebaceous-gland suppression tests, 81
  subacute toxicity tests, 81, 82
mutagenesis assessment, 101–106
  mammalian assay systems, 104–106
  NCI studies, 101
  sub-mammalian assay systems, 102–104
predictive tests, 124
various methods, 1
Sinus carcinomas,
  relation to drug exposure, 51
Skeletal-bone tumors,
  myelogenous leukemia,
    incidence in CRCD control rats, 9
  osteogenic sarcomas, 6, 7, 9, 51, 63
    incidence in CRCD control rats, 7, 9
    incidence in inbred mouse strains, 63
    incidence in wild mice, 63
    relation to drug exposure, 51
    spontaneous development in CRCD control rats, 6
  periosteal fibromas,
    incidence in Sprague-Dawley and Fischer rats, 58
Skeletal-muscle tumors,
  fibrosarcomas,
    incidence in CRCD control rats, 9
  rhabdomyosarcomas,
    incidence in Sprague-Dawley and Fischer rats, 58
Skin tumors,
  adenomas, 8, 57
    incidence in CRCD control rats, 8
    incidence in Sprague-Dawley and Fischer rats, 57
  carcinomas, 6–8, 51, 57, 60, 61, 64
    incidence in CRCD control rats, 7, 8
    incidence in inbred mouse strains, 60, 61, 64
    incidence in Sprague-Dawley and Fischer rats, 57
    relation to drug exposure, 51
    spontaneous development in CRCD control rats, 6

fibroadenomas, 6, 8
  incidence in CRCD control rats, 8
  spontaneous development in CRCD control rats, 6
keratoacanthomas, 6–8
  incidence in CRCD control rats, 7, 8
  spontaneous development in CRCD control rats, 6
lipomas,
  incidence in CRCD control rats, 8
papillomas, 6, 7, 60, 61, 64
  incidence in CRCD control rats, 7
  incidence in inbred mouse strains, 60, 61, 64
  spontaneous development in CRCD control rats, 6
sarcomas,
  relation to drug exposure, 51
trichoepitheliomas, 6, 7
  incidence in CRCD control rats, 7
  spontaneous development in CRCD control rats, 6
verruca vulgaris,
  incidence in Sprague-Dawley and Fischer rats, 57
Soft-tissue sarcomas,
  relation to drug exposure, 51
Somatic-cell assays,
  Chinese hamster, 104
  diploid human cells, 105
  mouse lymphoma, 104, 105
Spider monkey,
  lymphoma-virus susceptibility, 67
Splenic tumors,
  lymphomas, 6, 8
    incidence in CRCD control rats, 8
    spontaneous development in CRCD control rats, 6
  reticulum-cell sarcomas,
    incidence in CRCD control rats, 8
Spontaneous-tumor incidence,
  Chinese hamster, 65
  dogs, 65, 66
  Fischer rats, 57, 58
  influencing factors, 55, 56
    endocrine, 55
    environmental, 56
    immunologic, 55, 56
    nutritional, 55
  monkeys, 66, 67
  related pathologic changes, 55–68
  Sprague-Dawley rats, 56
  Syrian hamster, 65
  variation between control groups, 9
Squamous-cell carcinomas,
  incidence in CRCD control rats, 7, 8
  incidence in inbred mouse strains, 64
  incidence in Sprague-Dawley and Fischer rats, 57
  spontaneous development in CRCD control rats, 6
Squirrel monkey,
  lymphoma-virus susceptibility, 67
Statistical consideration in carcinogenic testing,
  benefits of larger numbers of test animals, 3
  biologic validity, 11
  comparison of tumor development in test and control
    animals, 3, 4
  correlation to biological findings, 11
  interpretation of results, 11
  "no effect" level, 4

number of surviving test animals, 1
  significance in extrapolation of animal data to man, 47
  threshold dose, 42, 43
  variation in incidence of spontaneous tumors, 3
Steroids, androgenic-anabolic,
  carcinogenic effect in man, 52
Stilbestrol,
  carcinogenic effects in man, 52
  therapeutic applications, 52
  tumorigenicity following prenatal exposure, 26
Streptozotocin,
  determination of mutagenicity, 85
Striated-muscle tumors,
  spontaneous development in CRCD control rats, 6
Stubtailed monkey,
  lymphoma-virus susceptibility, 67
Subacute toxicity tests, 81, 82
Sub-mammalian assay systems, 101–104
  metabolic conversions, 101
  Neurospora crassa ad-3 mutants, 103
  Rosenkranz prescreening test, 102
  Saccharomyces cerevisiae, 103
  Salmonella tester sets, 102
Sympathicoblastomas, endocrine,
  incidence in Sprague-Dawley and Fischer rats, 57
Syrian hamsters, inbred, 15

T

Teratogenic tests,
  lack of correlation for determining carcinogenic
     potential, 1
Teratomas,
  incidence in inbred mouse strains, 60, 61, 64
  incidence in wild mice, 64
Test animals,
  extrapolation of data to man, 45–47
    appropriate selection of test animal, 45
    assessment of statistical significance, 47
    metabolism of test compound, 46
    route of administration, 46
    transplacental administration of carcinogens, 46
  group size for positive controls, 30
  interpretation of test results in terms of carcinogenic
     potential, 41–43
  numbers suggested for studies, 3
  selection of species, 15
  selection of strains, 1–3, 15
  studies of carcinogenic responses, 48, 49
    effects of griseofulvin administration, 49
    effects of isoniazid administration, 48
    effects of metronidazole administration, 48
Testicular tumors,
  interstitial-cell tumors, 6, 8, 57, 60
    incidence in CRCD control rats, 8
    incidence in inbred mouse strains, 60
    incidence in Sprague-Dawley and Fischer rats, 57
    spontaneous development in CRCD control rats, 6
  teratomas,
    incidence in inbred mouse strains, 60, 61
Test results,

interpretation, 5–10, 41–43, 45–49
  in relation to test animals, 41–43
  in terms of significance to man, 45–49
  in relation to control animals, 5–10
  susceptibility of different species, 42
Tetradecanoyl phorbol acetate,
  tumor promotion, 39
(−)-*trans*-Δ^9-Tetrahydrocannabinol,
  use with virus, 86
Thorotrast,
  carcinogenic effect in man, 51
Threshold dose,
  biological threshold, 42
  dose–response relationship, 42
  statistical considerations, 42, 43
Thymic tumors,
  carcinomas, 6, 7
    incidence in CRCD control rats, 7
    spontaneous development in CRCD control rats, 6
  sarcomas, 6, 7
    incidence in CRCD control rats, 7
    spontaneous development in CRCD control rats, 6
  thymomas, 6, 8
    incidence in CRCD control rats, 8
    spontaneous development in CRCD control rats, 6
Thymidine-^{14}C,
  uptake into DNA, 105
Thymidine kinase,
  deficiency in mutant hamster cells, 104
Thymomas,
  incidence in CRCD control rats, 8
  spontaneous development in CRCD control rats, 6
Thyroid tumors,
  adenocarcinomas, 6, 8
    incidence in CRCD control rats, 8
    spontaneous development in CRCD control rats, 6
  adenomas, 6, 8, 57
    incidence in CRCD control rats, 8
    incidence in Sprague-Dawley and Fischer rats, 57
    spontaneous development in CRCD control rats, 6
Tissue-culture models, *see* Cell cultures
TK, *see* Thymidine kinase
Tobacco carcinogenesis, 35
TPA, *see* Tetradecanoyl phorbol acetate
Transitional-cell carcinomas,
  incidence in CRCD control rats, 7, 8
  spontaneous development in CRCD control rats, 6
Triazides,
  classification of chemical carcinogens, 80
Trichoepitheliomas,
  incidence in CRCD control rats, 7
  spontaneous development in CRCD control rats, 6
Tumor development,
  deficits in cell-mediated immunity, 19
  effect of environmental contaminants in control
    animals, 56
  effect of griseofulvin administration, 9, 10, 49
  effect of isoniazid administration, 48
  effect of metronidazole administration, 48
  esophageal, in hamsters, 29
  following prenatal exposure, 23, 25, 26
  influence of immunologic factors, 55, 56

inhibition by diet, 17
pathogenesis of observed effects, 42
reduction of latent period, 26, 55
  assessment of drug carcinogenicity, 55
  following prenatal exposure, 26
Tumorigens,
  definition, 41
Tumor initiators, 36, 37, 39
Tumor progression, 87
Tumor promoters, 36, 39
Tumors,
  definition, 41
Tumor transplants, 71

U

Uracil mustard,
  use as positive control compound, 31, 32
Ultraviolet radiation, 86, 87, 104
  effect on mutation in Chinese hamster cells, 104
  effect on xeroderma pigmentosum patients, 86
  levels of DNA repair synthesis in xeroderma pigmento-
    sum, 87
Urethane,
  carcinogenic activity, 81
  inhibition of carcinogenicity, 19
  transformation of neurofibrosarcoma cells, 115
  tumorigenicity following prenatal exposure, 25, 26
  use as positive control compound, 32
Urocystic tumors,
  carcinomas, 6–8, 51
    incidence in CRCD control rats, 7, 8
    relation to drug exposure, 51
    spontaneous development in CRCD control rats, 6
  epithelial hyperplasia, 81, 82
  papillomas, 57, 64
    incidence in inbred mouse strains, 64
    incidence in Sprague-Dawley and Fischer rats, 57
Uterine tumors,
  adenocarcinomas, 6, 7, 63
    incidence in CRCD control rats, 7
    incidence in inbred mouse strains, 63
    spontaneous development in CRCD control rats, 6
  leioyomas, 57, 63
    incidence in inbred mouse strains, 63
    incidence in Sprague-Dawley and Fischer rats, 57
  polyps, 6–8
    incidence in CRCD control rats, 7, 8
    spontaneous development in CRCD control rats, 6
  sarcomas, 6, 7, 63
    incidence in CRCD control rats, 7
    incidence in inbred mouse strains, 63

spontaneous development in CRCD control rats, 6

V

Vaginal tumors,
  adenocarcinomas,
    relation to drug exposure, 51
  leiomyosarcomas, 6, 7
    incidence in CRCD control rats, 7
    spontaneous development in CRCD control rats, 6
Verruca vulgaris,
  incidence in Sprague-Dawley and Fischer rats, 57
Viral activation,
  transformation of cell cultures, 92
Viruses,
  activation by chemicals, 86
  combined action with chemicals, 93
  stimulation of cells to form tumors, 83
Vitamin A,
  content in chow diets, 18
Vitamin A deficiency, dietary,
  effect on carcinogenesis in the colon, 18
Vitamin B_{12},
  content in chow diets, 18
  effect on toxicity and carcinogenicity of chemicals, 17
Vitamin D,
  content in chow diets, 18
von Recklinghausen's disease, 115

W

World Health Organization,
  recommended dosage levels, 3, 47
  report on testing and evaluation of drugs for carcino-
    genicity, 45

X

Xeroderma pigmentosum,
  DNA damage and repair, 86, 87
X-rays,
  effect on mutation in Chinese hamster cells, 104
  effect on mutation in diploid human cells, 105
  effect on mutation in mouse lymphoma cells, 105

Z

Zinc,
  content in chow diets, 18